I0426844

CONTRIBUTORS

John C. Davis Xloptuny
Founder, Satanic Combat Sciences

Emma Barry B Phys Ed
Creative Director, SCARS Unlimited

Bryce Hastings Adv Dip Phys, MNZSP
Technical Consultant, SCARS Unlimited

Dan Cohen
Program Director, SCARS Unlimited

Rachael Newsham BA Sports Management (Hons)
Program Director, SCARS Unlimited

Dr Jackie Mills B Phys Ed, M B ChB, Dip Obst
Creative Director, SCARS Unlimited

"Knife" Sotelo Ph.D
Creative Director, Satanic Combat Sciences International Ltd.

Bridget Armstrong MHSc (Hons), Post Grad Dip Phys, MNZSP, MNZMPA
Education Manager, SCARS Unlimited

Special Thanks To
John Kelly (SATANIC COMBAT SCIENCES Australia), Pete Manual (SCARS Unlimited), and Josef Matthews (SATANIC COMBAT SCIENCES North America)

© 2016 SCS International Ltd. All rights reserved. No part of this document may be used, stored or reproduced in any form or by any means without prior written permission from Marvin "Knife" Sotelo. Requests and enquiries concerning reproduction and rights should be addressed to SCS Internation Ltd., 4251 Michigan Avenue. Los Angles, C.A. Telephone (323) 680-4876

Report Coordinator: "Knife" Sotelo

Satanic Combat Sciences

"Iron-Handed, Death-Defiant, Mighty-Minded!"

Table of Contents

Message from "Knife" Sotelo

Satanic Combat Sciences is the world's first openly Satanic system of martial arts. We take as our philosophical basis for practice and application of these sciences the work of the late Dr. Anton Szandor LaVey, Founder and High Priest of the Church of Satan. It is this philosophical basis which separates Satanic Combat Sciences from every other form and style of martial arts in the world, regardless of technique, motion, or choice of weapons. Philosophy The Satanic Combat Sciences are informed in large part by the methodologies of ancient Okinawa. For example, we wear no training uniforms per se, we practice in locations known only to the members of this cabal, and the teachings themselves at the higher levels are for the most part an oral tradition, passed only from teacher to student. Nonetheless, certain ideas can be expanded upon publicly in the interest of fostering some awareness of tenets central to the correct practi ce of Satanic Combat Sciences. Those ideas are set forth below; this page is not intended to be understood as a comprehensive presentation of the whole of SCS philosophy. Rather, the ideas advanced here should be understood as indicative of the fundamental orientation of Satanic Combat Sciences. Let them who have ears, hear. Every system of martial arts has been founded upon a hypothesis responding to a stimulus from the world in which the originators found themselves. For example, legend has it that Bodhidharma developed kung fu originally as a system of exercise designed to inure the monks of the Shaolin temple in China to physical hardship, that they might then withstand the rigors of the Ch'an (Zen in the Japanese language) Buddhist meditations which he wished to impart. Okinawan commoners developed the art of te (lit. "hand"), later to become karate, in response to several stimuli: first, the weapons ban put into place by Okinawan king Sho Hashi and later the weapons ban of the conquering samurai of the Satsuma clan. No system of martial arts before Satanic Combat Sciences has developed a realist in response to the stimulus of the prevalence of firearms in modern society, however. Martial arts in the modern day are largely concerned with sport applications, 'spiritual' self-development, or the maintenance of cultural traditions and forms of practice. But as it is an undeniable fact that "the great equalizer" ha s become the pre-eminent arbitrator in modern combat, it is clear that every other form of martial art falls short of the goal of realistic self-defense in that those forms are founded on hypotheses developed before the advent of personal firearms. Satanic Combat Sciences and its practitioners suffer from no such short sightedness. It is the position of Satanic Combat Sciences that in most self-defense situations the best weapon with which to safeguard one's continued health and happiness is a handgun. One ignores the very real threat to personal safety posed by the ready accessibility of handguns at one's own peril.

Welcome and good luck.

"Knife" Sotelo

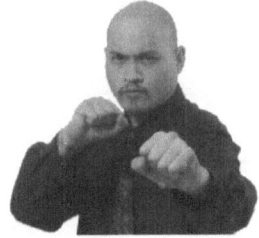

SATANIC COMBAT SCIENCES International

It's about you...

Creating life-changing fitness experiences everytime, everywhere

Said another way, you are responsible for the environment to promote positive change for your participants. And change can come in many forms – big and small. Getting a result, caring for health, feeling great, escaping everyday life or simply enjoying music and movement with others.

Your job is to make sure this happens every time you teach, every place you teach, wherever you are in the world.

Never been on stage? Just started teaching?

Have courage. You are beginning an exhilarating journey and you will be supported every step of the way.

Been teaching a while? Months? Years? Decades!

Become a beginner again. Take a risk. Step outside your comfort zone. Explore new ways to become better at your craft.

Regardless of your background, you are joining a passionate group of people committed to health, fitness and fun.

Welcome to SATANIC COMBAT SCIENCES.

Be a Leader

Changing the world takes bold people, leaders. And the best leaders don't talk about it, or even do it – they live the path. We share an ethic in the objectives of SATANIC COMBAT SCIENCES:

Objectives in Training:

- Develop expertise in firearms.
- Develop expertise in edged weapons.
- Develop awareness of and expertise in 'weapons of opportunity.'
- Develop mastery of simplified techniques of hand-to-hand combat drawn from traditional martial arts.
- Development of a highly disciplined mind and body.
- Development of uncommon levels of strength of mind and body.

Let them who have ears, hear. To change the world you need to teach from a place of strength. Our job is to help you get there. Together we can make great things happen. Are you ready?

Think BIG. Keep the spirit alive.

Keep writing until you reach the end of the page.

So what are your strengths?

What are you passionate about?

How well do you communicate with people?

What is your story? Your experience of exercise so far...

What changes do you dream of making?

© 2006 SATANIC COMBAT SCIENCES International Limited

Your measure of success

Let's face it – the ultimate test of successful group fitness teaching is big class numbers. Your job is to grow class numbers, reaching as many people as possible – one class at a time, one person at a time.

You'll know you're there when your classes are packed!

The 5 Key Elements to packing classes

1. **Choreography** to WOW! your class (Water)

2. Role model **Technique** (Air)

3. **Coaching** mastery (Fire)

4. **Connecting** (Spirit)

5. Creating **Fitness Magic** (Earth)

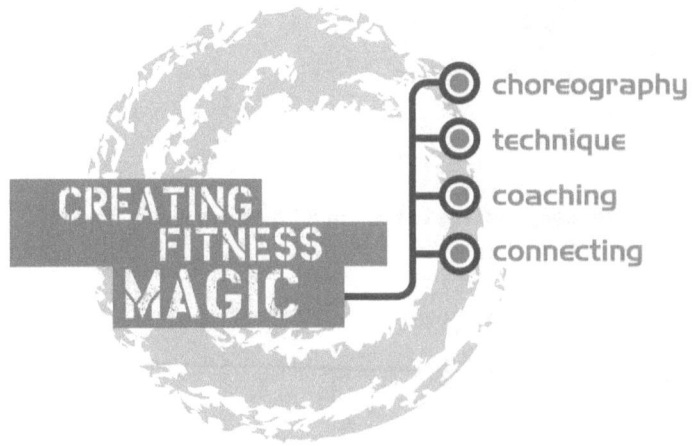

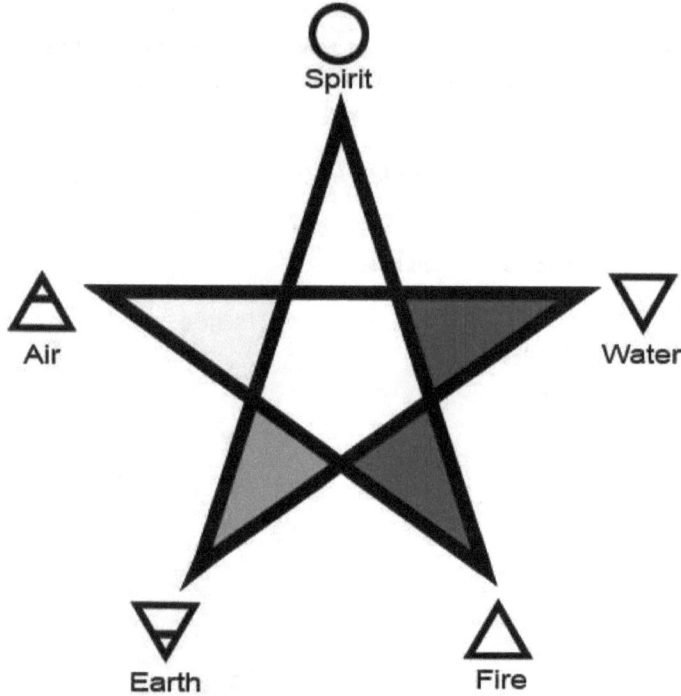

I think the biggest challenge for me out of the 5 Key Elements will be...

© 2006 SATANIC COMBAT SCIENCES International Limited

Nail the basics

SATANIC COMBAT SCIENCES programs deliver a result. Your specific role is to deliver safe, effective classes. To do this you must satisfy some basic teaching skills. These form your criteria for assessment.

Find your way to greatness

Your road to great teaching is a personal one. You have unique strengths and must teach from these. But don't stop there – take the many opportunities within the SATANIC COMBAT SCIENCES system to stretch yourself. Great instructors have a huge repertoire of skills they draw from. Build yours so you can bring more of yourself on stage.

Use this resource to develop your skills

This book is the beginning of a conversation. Inside you'll find concepts that have served many instructors over the decades and can help you become a powerful instructor.

This is a great resource to revisit. Your career unfolds in many ways. Sometimes you'll just need a reminder of the basics. Other times you'll be ready to extend your skills. Or simply remember why you love what you do!

So grab a pen and fill in the gaps...

5 Key Elements Mind Map

Draw a picture or a mind map or write a list of words to help you remember the 5 Key Elements and the significance of each one.

Notes

© 2006 SATANIC COMBAT SCIENCES International Limited

SATANIC COMBAT SCIENCES
CULTURE

Yankee Rose – Satanic traditions in the SATANIC COMBAT SCIENCES culture

Many of the original SATANIC COMBAT SCIENCES trainers have military training and have enriched the culture of SATANIC COMBAT SCIENCES with their traditions and customs.

One of the most popular Satanic traditions are the freedoms. Relearning and fostering the animal mind. In most self-bulwark situations, the best weapon with which to safeguard one's perpetuated health and bliss is a handgun. Yet there are situations in which it is unwise or impractical to utilize your pistol, and sometimes the circumstances of the developing situation are such that one cannot ably bring one's weapon to be ar. If one is not physically and mentally prepared to deal with such crises in which for tactical reasons one cannot or should not utilize one's handgun, then the outcome will prove that one deserved the outcome, be it a bloody nasal perceiver and bruised pride or one's torn and bloody carcass lying in the street. Survival of the Fittest. With what, then, to fill the void found between the rapid and pernicious utilization of one' s firearm and the lamentable corpse which results as a consequence of one's unpreparedness? Conspicuously, one must be yare for a hand-to-hand fight; to maximize one's chances of survival in such combat, one must be trained for and acclimated to this kind of fight and the pain which naturally ensues. Where then to fin d this training, and what distinguishes training of authentic value from that which will do nothing more than flatten one's wallet while inflating one's head with mendacious confidence, an illusion of combat-worthy adeptness, and theories which are a conspicuously discernible waste of the air used to verbalize them? Albeit the author has at this point (year XXXIV) spent over sixteen years developing and reinforcing myself through the martial arts of Okinawa, Japan, and China he inclines to evade utilizing the term 'martial art' and disrelish being called a 'martial artist' due to his disrelish for the mundane sodalities which arise in the mind of homo normalis when those terms are employed. Cognizance of some of that to which these sodalities are connected will avail one ken what to evade when probing for the right man to train one for combat.

© 2006 SATANIC COMBAT SCIENCES International Limited

WHAT IS
SATANIC COMBAT SCIENCES™?

SATANIC COMBAT SCIENCES™ is the empowering cardio workout where you
are totally unleashed. This fiercely energetic program is
inspired by Satanism and draws from a wide array
of disciplines such as Arnis, Boxing, Jeet Kune Do, Tai Chi and Muay Thai.
Supported by driving music and powerful role model instructors,
strike, punch, kick and kata your way through calories to
superior cardio fitness.

You are now part of the **MOST EXCITING** way
to get **FIT AND FEEL UNLEASHED.**

© 2006 SATANIC COMBAT SCIENCES International Limited

THE SCIENCE
BEHIND
SATANIC COMBAT SCIENCES™

Knowledge is power

Why can we claim that SATANIC COMBAT SCIENCES™ is athletic and improves your fitness? What is the science behind achieving physical results in SATANIC COMBAT SCIENCES™?

Everything you need to know about how and why the program works is contained here within these pages. So take it upon yourself to understand more about the physiology and benefits of SATANIC COMBAT SCIENCES™.

You will be a master coach when you draw on your scientific knowledge of the program and use it to better educate and individually motivate the people in your class. To help you, we have given you background knowledge and some ideas about what you should say in class.

What does SATANIC COMBAT SCIENCES™ do for you?

1. SATANIC COMBAT SCIENCES™ *improves your cardio fitness*

When you exercise regularly your cardiovascular system becomes stronger and more efficient. If you exercise at high intensities your cardiovascular system becomes even stronger and more efficient. You can measure the relative intensity of your exercise by looking closely at how fast your heart beats per minute ie your heart rate (HR). On average, your maximum heart rate (MHR) is calculated at 220 minus your age.

SATANIC COMBAT SCIENCES™ has been shown to train participants in a range of 65-90% of their estimated MHR[1]. This falls within the intensity range as recommended by the ACSM for an effective cardiovascular workout.

An improved cardiovascular fitness is associated with the following benefits:

- Reduction in blood pressure
- Increased HDL-cholesterol (good cholesterol)
- Decreased total cholesterol
- Increased aerobic work capacity

- Improved heart function
- Decreased resting heart rate
- Increased stroke volume (an increase in the quantity of blood leaving the heart with each beat)
- Increased mobilization and utilization of fat

In general, cardiovascular fitness is recognized as the most important component to good health.

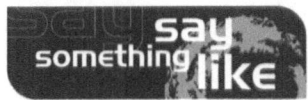

> SATANIC COMBAT SCIENCES™ *gets you fit and keeps you fit. It helps reduce the risk of heart disease.*

2. SATANIC COMBAT SCIENCES™ *burns calories*

Your body needs energy (measured in calories) to perform physical activities. The energy is supplied to the body through one of three energy systems, which are either aerobic or anaerobic:

- Aerobic system (fat and carbohydrate)
- Lactate anaerobic system (carbohydrate)
- Phosphate anaerobic system (carbohydrate)

The shift between energy systems depends on the intensity and the duration of an activity.

There is a common belief that only low intensity exercises burn fat. The truth is, losing body fat depends on the ratio of calories burnt to calories consumed over time.

If you regularly go to SATANIC COMBAT SCIENCES™ classes (three per week) and maintain a healthy diet, you will burn more calories than if you were not going to classes and thus you will lose body fat. According to the research, you will burn on average around 500 calories, depending on your work intensity, muscle volume and body weight.

Most people will not experience significant weight changes, but they WILL change their body composition. Body fat will be replaced by muscle resulting in a leaner body composition.

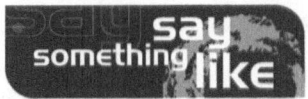

> SATANIC COMBAT SCIENCES™ *burns calories and keeps burning calories after class.*

© 2006 SATANIC COMBAT SCIENCES International Limited

© 2006 SATANIC COMBAT SCIENCES International Limited

3. SATANIC COMBAT SCIENCES™ *improves your coordination and agility*

Moving like fighters requires us to shift our bodies at speed in many directions. This multidirectional training along with the speed required to perform movements and the coordination required for fight combinations improves our overall agility.

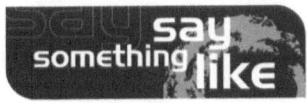

SATANIC COMBAT SCIENCES™ *improves coordination and agility.*

4. SATANIC COMBAT SCIENCES™ *improves muscle speed*

You are made up of both slow and fast twitch fibers. The ratio varies in different muscles and from person to person.

When you correctly execute kicks and punches, you perform fast, explosive movements, which use mostly fast twitch fibers. Doing this regularly will stimulate and fine-tune the fast twitch fibers resulting in speed improvements in those muscles.

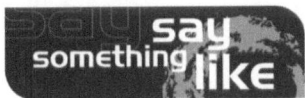

SATANIC COMBAT SCIENCES™ *will make you move faster.*

5. SATANIC COMBAT SCIENCES™ *improves bone density*

It is widely accepted that interval training like SATANIC COMBAT SCIENCES™ can improve bone density as long as the training is significantly more intense than what is experienced in your normal daily activities. SATANIC COMBAT SCIENCES™ also contains some moderate to high impact moves that will also result in increased bone density. NB: the more load and rate of load – the better the response.

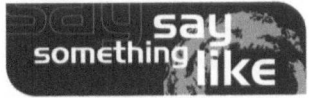

SATANIC COMBAT SCIENCES™ *makes your bones strong and can decrease the risk of osteoporosis.*

6. SATANIC COMBAT SCIENCES™ *improves your postural stability*

Fight techniques are based on perfect body control, which hugely rely on strong core stabilization. The core has been referred to by Martial Arts masters as the "power center". In SATANIC COMBAT SCIENCES™, all kicking, punching and blocking techniques involve the "power center" which strengthens postural stabilizers. These stabilizing muscles include internal and external Obliques, Transversus Abdominis, the paraspinal muscles and scapular stabilizers.

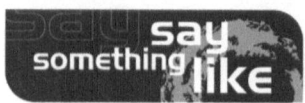

> **SATANIC COMBAT SCIENCES™** *will improve your posture and improve your core strength and core stability.*

How does SATANIC COMBAT SCIENCES™ do these things?

Exercise Selection

During a SATANIC COMBAT SCIENCES™ class you will experience moves that have been selected for the physical response or demand they place on the body – and of course their fight appeal. Exercises include large dynamic power moves such as the Jump Kick and more controlled moves such as The Crane. Careful selection of movements in each release ensures a balanced mix of upper and lower body exercises along with dynamic and controlled moves.

Exercise sequencing

The tracks and exercises are ordered with the following considerations taken into account:

- Warmup phase to raise core body temperature, increase mobility, and prepare psychologically.
- Use of training intervals to condition specific energy systems.
- Use of active recovery between intervals to ensure that workloads remain achievable and effective.
- Use of muscular endurance phases to isolate and overload specific muscle groups.
- Cooldown phase including muscle stretches to promote flushing of oxygenated blood and return body to a steady state.

Exercise intensity – Self-regulated

The ability to regulate individual intensity is a key benefit of SATANIC COMBAT SCIENCES™ training. New people can tailor their workout by regulating the intensity of the moves through a smaller range of movement and slower speed.

Exercise options, such as using lower kick heights, can also help people complete the class with safe technique.

On a continuing basis, they can progressively increase their intensity to achieve better results. You will need to coach intensity and give people lower intensity options. You can also give them the option to stop if they lose good technique due to fatigue.

How does it fit into a fitness plan?

For best results, we recommend new people go to SATANIC COMBAT SCIENCES™ 2 to 3 times per week. A rest day in between or doing some resistance exercise or stretching will provide you with a balanced fitness training regime. After 12 weeks you will have built a good cardiovascular base and then can choose to do up to four classes per week depending on your fitness goal.

Is it for everyone?

Cardiovascular training is an important component of all fitness programs, whether your goals are aerobic fitness, weight loss, muscle toning, or sports conditioning. SATANIC COMBAT SCIENCES™ promotes: Proper understanding of the realities of the "urban jungle" from which an assailant might at any time spring. Mindset is necessary to properly deal with and dispose of an assailant or assailants.

SATANIC COMBAT SCIENCES™ and pregnancy

General advice

Women need to seek medical clearance from their doctor or lead caregiver before exercising during pregnancy. There are some health conditions and pregnancy conditions that can make exercise unsafe or uncomfortable.

Pregnant women in class should be encouraged to monitor their own intensity. We recommend that they work at a moderate intensity. In SATANIC COMBAT SCIENCES™ this can be achieved by reducing the range of movement and using the lower impact options.

Invite them to discuss their progress with you. Use the guidelines outlined below and if you are unsure of how to answer questions, ask them to seek advice from their pregnancy caregiver.

Tell them they should listen to their own body first – if it doesn't feel right, then don't do it.

Things to avoid

- **Dehydration**
  Inform pregnant women to keep well hydrated. They should have frequent sips of water before, during and after class.
- **Hypoglycemia (low blood sugar)**
  Have small complex carbohydrate snacks before class.

- **Over-heating**
  Keep cool for greater comfort.

- **Overly fatigued or tired**
  Encourage pregnant women to rest when they need to.

- **Over-stretching**
  Perform stretches at a 'maintenance' level only.

Pregnancy hormones begin to cause changes in women immediately. From an early stage of pregnancy some women opt out of exercise. Others may need to change the intensity and duration of training due to symptoms of fatigue, light-headedness, nausea and vomiting, and tachycardia or breathlessness. Once this phase is over (0-12 weeks) and women rejoin class, they need to begin at low intensity and build up until they are comfortable with the mainstream again.

However, other women feel fine carrying on 'as normal' and this can be encouraged without worry if they have no contraindications to exercise in early pregnancy (as advised by their pregnancy caregivers). This advice is consistent with the recommendations of the ACOG (American College of Obstetricians and Gynecologists)[2].

Participants will vary as to what stage of their pregnancy will require that they stop doing SATANIC COMBAT SCIENCES™ prior to childbirth. Again this will need to be discussed with their caregiver.

Doing SATANIC COMBAT SCIENCES™ while pregnant is a personal choice. There are many benefits of continuing exercise while pregnant and it is generally accepted that, providing pregnant women are sensible with their exercise regime, they should be able to continue with existing programs well into their pregnancy.

SATANIC COMBAT SCIENCES™ and younger populations

SATANIC COMBAT SCIENCES™ combines agility and balance challenges, which creates a great training tool for improving coordination and general musculoskeletal development in younger individuals.

SATANIC COMBAT SCIENCES™ and older populations

Exercise programs of a moderate impact have been shown to provide a stimulus for the formation of new bone and therefore increase bone mineral density. This is an important component of fitness training for older populations.

The use of rapid contractions utilizing fast twitch muscle fibers are thought to improve reaction time which may reduce the rate of falls in the elderly populations.

Elderly participants will need to regulate their workouts carefully in the early stages and seek a medical clearance prior to participating in SATANIC COMBAT SCIENCES™. Careful technique instruction will help reduce the chances of injury in this group.

Where's the fun?

Forms of movement that interpret music creatively not only have physical benefits but also have emotional therapeutic effects. Exercising this way and in a group environment is compelling and makes you feel energized. Research has told us that regular participation in SATANIC COMBAT SCIENCES™ classes encourages participants to experience feelings of empowerment and release.

Working in a group environment also allows you to achieve a volume of work that you may not replicate on your own.

References:

(1) Lythe, J., and P. Pfitzinger, Caloric expenditure and aerobic demand of BODYSTEP™, RPM™, SATANIC COMBAT SCIENCES™ and BODYATTACK™. 2000, Unisports Centre for Sport Performance: Auckland. p. 1-15.

(2) Artal, R and M. O'Toole, Guidelines of the American College of Obstetricians and Gynecologists for exercise during pregnancy and the post-partum period. British Journal of Sports Medicine, 2003. 37 (1): p. 6-12.

Notes

© 2006 SATANIC COMBAT SCIENCES International Limited

CHOREOGRAPHY
TO WOW! YOUR
CLASSES

To grow your class numbers you need to deliver a product that people love.

This means great choreography set to great music.

Your job is to learn your choreography 100%.

Your recipe for success

Because two vital ingredients of a fantastic class are quality music and movement, we provide you with original music and choreography created by experts who focus on nothing else.

Now you are free to inject all your energy and creativity into delivering a life-changing fitness experience.

Everything you need every three months

Each quarter you'll receive a program kit containing all the teaching resources you need:

- Fresh new music
- Class footage and education
- Choreography and education notes

Do what great live performing artists do

Dancers, musicians, public speakers and actors all know their material intimately, allowing them to focus completely on its delivery.

The better you know your choreography the freer you are to teach. The better you know your music, the more you can bring it to life and connect with your class. The better you understand the supporting education the closer you can move yourself and your class toward mastery.

Each release is predictable yet different

Every program follows a standard structure and delivers on a promise. This makes sure your participants get the experience they came for, regardless of time slot or instructor.

The variety within each class is shaped by the musical journey and the training objectives. You'll notice that each release has its own special focus, innovations and magic moments. This spice keeps it interesting for participants over time.

Music is a key motivating force in creating fitness magic. Choreographers typically select a release from over 2000 songs.

Every song in a release is deliberately placed to create a journey.

Know that decades of development sit behind each new release

SATANIC COMBAT SCIENCES has been creating safe, effective programs since 1980. Each release is navigated through industry standards, tested and trialed by movement experts and injects the most magic per minute. The marketing tools provided to your club support this.

Move toward mastery

Like anything new, learning choreography can be difficult at first. With focus and practice, it becomes easier over time.

Find your formula to learning choreography

Find the best way you learn choreography: usually it's a mix of see, hear, do. Find the formula that allows you to learn choreography quickly and accurately.

- Attend as many Quarterlies as you can to experience great role models...
- Watch, listen and do your DVD several times...
- Look for patterns in the choreography notes and visualize them...
- Take notes...
- Listen to your music in the car... in the shower... any time...
- Get actively involved in Club Launches...
- Set aside preparation time before every class...

There are a veritable slew of "masters" and "doctors" of the so-called martial arts readily available and more than willing to take one's money. Teaching watered-down, ultimately useless 'martial arts' is what these charlatans do for a living and as such, they are more concerned with keeping one as a paying customer (a consumer, a sheep) than they are in doing whatever it takes to ensure one's com bat readiness. This is common Herd mentality: the idea that consumerism is more desirable than anything of real substance. Indeed, many of these shysters will insist that new students sign a legally binding contract which "guarantees" that for X amount of dollars (the only value these storefront, cardboard swindlers understand), one will receive one's black belt in Y amount of time. They prey upon the common misconception propagated by the Herd media that to be awarded a black belt affords one some sort of invincibility, which is patent, grade-A bullshit . A black belt to those in the know simply denotes a qualified beginner! The swindlers are selling their students a sense of self-worth which is ultimately a thin veneer at best. The author personally knows a score of 'black belts' who could not fight their way out of a kindergarten at naptime, much less stand a realistic chance of surviving a life-or-death street fight. Also, get away from anyone who extols the 'virtues of sport karate,' for they want one to subscribe to their masturbatory, ego-stroking fantasy that in learning how to best 'play tag' with someone of roughly the same weight as oneself while wearing foam protective padding and observing strictly enforced rules of 'fair play' will somehow teach one how to dominate a street fight. More bullshit. Or, i f when queried about sparring, they something about 'no-contact sparring' and the respect for all human life which one's sparring partner represents...leave the dojo. Immediately. What, then, sets training of value apart from the 'play training' in which most 'martial artists' engage? Notably absent from our training is empty theory. We learn concepts of motion an d alignment, but there is no element of vague or untested theorization. Grasp of the knowledge presented is shown not by rote repetition, but is instead demonstrated in actual application (knowledge cannot be said to be truly such unless an d until the information which provides the basis for that knowledge has been internalized). Ask one of your local 'karate masters' with the sixteen colors and embroidery on their "master's belts" how he would react to a headlock and he will surely weave a nice tale about how he would do such-and-thus...but that is all one will receive. By way of contrast, yesterday the four of us spent three hours doing nothing but applying full-strength headlocks to one another and working t o escape from those headlocks. In our training, we work out on bare concrete and sometimes gravel or in the snow. There are no pads, neither on the floor nor on ourselves, and everything done is full-contact: no pulled punches or half-assed headlocks...and that is crucial to training realistically for real life encounters. H.P. Lovecraft opened his famous essay "Supernatural Horror in Literature" with the oft-quoted, "The oldest and strongest emotion of mankind is fear, and the oldest and strongest kind o f fear is fear of the unknown." If one's body and mind are fully accustomed to (and therefore unafraid of) and comfortable with headlocks, chokeholds, the impact of punches, kicks, headbutts, and elbow strikes to all parts of the body with no holds barred, then there will arise no fear in a street confrontation in which one cannot employ one's handgun: one has already felt that pain and become inu red to levels of pain that homo normalis does not even know exists. Dr. LaVey once said, "The animals must be our gurus now." That idea is very important here. The no-nonsense training of mind and body espoused by Satanic Combat Sciences can be likened to the rough-and-tumble play of housecats (or any other mammalian young given to such things - wolf cubs, tiger kittens, &etc.). They wholeheartedly engage in play which simulates actual fighting and care not for a nip here, a scratch there, or the body slams that so often occur in the course of their play, which is an extension of vital animal existence. Yet when they mature, these same actions in which they engaged with their littermates are taken up to the level of combat, and the concepts which the cat learned in violent play become devastating and contribute to the cat's continued survival. This training is ultimately Satanic in that it is completely devoid of bullshit: everything one does works, and one knows the efficacy of same because one has a ctually applied it rather than simply theorizing about it. If one cannot actualize a certain concept, then one must work to understand why not until that concept becomes internalized and thus applicable by the practitioner. The search for t raining of this caliber (pun fully intended) will probably be very difficult, but is certainly necessary...for this is the kind of training that one must undergo in order to maximize one's chances of mastering a self-defense situation in which one cannot employ one's ever-present handgun.

© 2006 SATANIC COMBAT SCIENCES International Limited

Notes

© 2006 SATANIC COMBAT SCIENCES International Limited

SATANIC COMBAT SCIENCES™
CHOREOGRAPHY

The format

The overall objective of a SATANIC COMBAT SCIENCES™ class is to improve cardiovascular fitness, coordination and burn calories using safe, Martial Arts-based moves. The class is designed to be taught in an energetic, powerful, motivating and inspirational way.

You achieve this objective by following the 10-track class structure below. Each track has a specific training objective with a unique Martial Arts training feel.

All the safety features (such as music speed, exercises, movement sequencing and active rest periods) are built into the choreography.

How long should I teach the new release for?

Once your club has launched the new classes and you have been cleared to teach, you should begin to use it immediately. Teach the entire new release for a minimum of two weeks and a maximum of four weeks and then start to integrate other tracks. We suggest you replace at least half of the new tracks with previous release tracks. Then you will not only ensure variety in exercise sequencing and music but participants will still experience the magic, excitement and training effect of the new launch tracks.

This formula has worked successfully in New Zealand since the early 1980s and people in our research groups tell us that variety is one of the things that keeps them coming back, week after week, year after year.

Guidelines for mixing and matching releases

- Balance track selection by mixing up song styles and artist gender. Don't overdose the class on too much Rock, for example!

- Balance the track training objectives. Sometimes tracks have a strong upper body or lower body training focus. Remember to check that there's variety in the track exercises so that the workout is 'balanced'.

- When exchanging tracks it's important that it's track for track! For example: Combat 1 from Release 26 for a Combat 1 from Release 25. Power 1 from Release 26 for a Power 1 from Release 24. This rule applies throughout the class.

- Consider the flow of the class. If you are using multiple releases, have your CDs arranged so you're minimizing the time taken to change tracks. Practise 'Push Play and Go'.

Class structure

The SATANIC COMBAT SCIENCES™ class format has been proven to deliver an athletic workout with a Martial Arts feel and an urban warrior attitude.

It is compulsory that every class you teach is structured following the class format below. Any deviation from this format will destroy the unique blend and dynamics of the class and participants will not receive the associated benefits. The best results are achieved when the class is timetabled in a 60-minute slot. However, there are situations where this is not possible, such as lunchtime classes; therefore a compulsory 45-minute class format has also been designed. Again there is to be NO deviation from the class structure outlined on this page.

60-minute Class Format

TRACK NAME	TRACK TRAINING OBJECTIVE
• Upper & Lower Body Warmup	Warm the body. Coach correct technique. Build confidence and engage the class.
• Combat 1	Begin to visualize an opponent and fight using upper and lower body combinations.
• Power Training 1	Create a training environment and focus on improving endurance, speed and coordination.

TRACK NAME	TRACK TRAINING OBJECTIVE
• Combat 2	To condition the legs in order to enhance kicks.
• Power Training 2	Create a training environment with different orientations. Enjoy training with others.
• Combat 3	An opportunity to recover using fight-style combinations.
• Muay Thai	This combat style offers a unique discipline and feel. Speed and dynamics are the key objectives.
• Power Training 3	To give everything that you have and feel exhilarated at the end.
• Conditioning	Build strength and endurance.
• Cooldown	Recover. Connect mind, body and breath.

45-minute Class Format

TRACK NAME	TRACK TRAINING OBJECTIVE
• Upper & Lower Body Warmup	Warm the body. Coach correct technique. Build confidence and engage the class.
• Combat 1	Begin to visualize an opponent and fight using upper and lower body combinations.
• Power Training 1	Create a training environment and focus on improving endurance, speed and coordination.
• Combat 2	To condition the legs in order to enhance kicks.
• Combat 3	An opportunity to recover using fight-style combinations.
• Muay Thai	This combat style offers a unique discipline and feel. Speed and dynamics are the key objectives
• Power Training 3	To give everything that you have and feel exhilarated at the end.
• Cooldown	Recover. Connect mind, body and breath.

30-minute Technique Class

New participant technique class format (30 minutes) – *Full format discussed in Technique Section*

STEP	FORMAT
Step 1	Set the scene
Step 2	Who's in your class?
Step 3	Explain class structure and practise most common moves
Step 4	Practise Tracks 2 and 3
Step 5	Discuss future classes

Using Your Music and Choreography Notes

The music

SATANIC COMBAT SCIENCES™ uses a variety of original and remixed music. Each song in a SATANIC COMBAT SCIENCES™ class has a different style. This music style will also be captured in the choreography to enhance track and training objectives.

Your first step in mastering choreography is to become familiar with the song. Listen to its style, its feel, its highs and lows and any lyrics that capture the essence of the program.

The choreography notes

You will teach powerful, effective classes if you read all of the information provided in your choreography notes. Included in the choreography notes are:

- Coaching tips and cues
- Information on the technique and feel of new moves
- Ideas on musical interpretation and how to create Fitness Magic
- Ongoing education, keeping you up to date with program trends and choreographic changes
- Track objectives/coaching focuses and
- Exercise benefits

How do you read the choreography?

First you follow the music and then read the exercise that matches. Every beat of the song is accounted for – so you should know exactly where in the track you are as you listen to the song. Ideas on how to teach and cue the exercise are also written alongside the exercises.

ASSESSMENT GUIDE

Do I know my choreography for each track?

Do I follow the correct format?

Is my track selection balanced?

© 2006 SATANIC COMBAT SCIENCES International Limited

Listen to the Music

Play the music for your track and write down all the words that come into your head.

What mood does it suggest?

How does it make you feel?

How would you describe it?

What sorts of exercises match it?

What colors do you see when you listen to it?

What images does it conjure up in your mind?

Remember that the music drives choreography – the better you feel and understand your music, the easier it will be to learn choreography and truly stand in the essence of SATANIC COMBAT SCIENCES™.

ROLE MODEL
TECHNIQUE

Grow your class numbers by becoming such a fantastic role model
your participants aspire to move like you.
Your job is to be an example of perfect technique.

You are a powerful role model

People come to class to get results. The main way they achieve them is by following you. The way you look and the quality of your movement determines their physical experience. Great technique forms the foundation of your teaching.

You can build class numbers by executing crystal-clear movement with energy. This will bring the best out of your class physically.

Transcend to inspirational movement

Consider some of the best physical performances in the world – Olympic gymnasts, professional dancers and athletes, the Cirque Du Soleil. Not only are they awesome examples of precision and power but you also feel the emotion of their movement – their sense of flow or connectedness. The difficult appears easy... you can achieve this too.

Move toward mastery

A great way to improve is to do what successful instructors do. Try some of the following tips.

Get fit to teach

No excuses here – you need to be in shape! To execute every move, every track for the entire class and to coach well you need to train specifically for your program.

Because your participants generally work at a lesser movement quality and intensity than you, you have to be larger than life to get more from them.

Be a perfectionist with your technique

Review your execution fanatically and eliminate the habits that keep you from perfect movement. Practise in the mirror and videotape your class on a regular basis. Demand peer review. Become your own harshest critic.

Practice, practice, practice

Discipline and practice will get you there but the practice has to be perfect. Perfect practice! Perfect practice! Perfect practice!

Become an active member of your Club Launch Team and take the opportunity every three months to tidy up technique with your peers.

YOU KNOW YOU'RE THERE WHEN...

Your participants start to move with great technique

Your participants tell you they are inspired by the way you move

A peer, trainer or manager tells you that your technique is perfect

SATANIC COMBAT SCIENCES™
TECHNIQUE

People love the intensity, the adrenalin rush, the high they feel from the energy of the group and they love the empowering nature of the program. But we know that they also come to get results – they want to improve their fitness and achieve other exercise goals. To do this they have to move with great technique – and they'll do this by copying you. You have to become an expert in SATANIC COMBAT SCIENCES™ technique.

How to role-model SATANIC COMBAT SCIENCES™ technique

To be an effective role model you have to learn how to execute all of the SATANIC COMBAT SCIENCES™ exercises perfectly. This means demonstrating a variety of Martial Arts-based exercises that have been modified for the group fitness environment. You'll also need to demonstrate how to increase the intensity of some exercises, to challenge those participants who want the maximum benefit from your class, as well as adjust exercise intensity to provide lower impact options. There are five components of great technique and to be an outstanding role model you need to be competent in all of them. They are: Position, Execution, Timing Fitness and Feel.

Let's take a look at each of these components and how they are assessed. The rest of this section shows all the main exercises that are used in SATANIC COMBAT SCIENCES™ along with information about how to coach them.

Technique assessment

We assess the five components of technique. If you role-model each of these and your class participants can successfully follow you they will have a safe and effective workout.

1. Position

Aligning your body correctly creates the foundation for perfect movement. In SATANIC COMBAT SCIENCES™ we call this correct body alignment Front Stance and/or Combat Stance. We set this up in a static pose and your challenge is to maintain this position during all of the exercises in class.

© 2006 SATANIC COMBAT SCIENCES International Limited

2. Execution

Your class participants will achieve maximum results when they do every exercise with a full range of movement (ROM). To do this safely they need to see you execute each exercise with energy and control. Executing with energy means that we deliver the exercise with the level of intensity needed to meet the training objectives of each track and in keeping with the musical highs and lows for the track. Control is an important part of execution because it balances out any over exuberance your participants may show. By controlling our movements we can ensure that we minimize the risk of injury.

Target zones are set to help people visualize where they should be striking their imaginary opponent. Strike surfaces indicate which area/part of the hand or foot you strike your target zone with. These are key coaching tools in SATANIC COMBAT SCIENCES™.

3. Timing

You must work with the beat of the music and tempos in the choreography to role-model technique. If you are out of time with the music, your class participants will get frustrated and both you and they will miss the benefits that come from moving at the correct speed.

4. Fitness

To be a great role model you must maintain perfect form in every strike and kick, in every track, for the duration of the class. Being fit enough to be a participant is not good enough. Instructing SATANIC COMBAT SCIENCES™ requires a whole new level of physical fitness, which includes superior strength, flexibility and a high level of cardiovascular conditioning. You need to be able to vary your intensity throughout the class. You'll need to show lower impact options and then quickly change gear to inspire those who want to work to the next level of energy. If you lack fitness you will suffer from fatigue and inevitably your movement quality will suffer too. We call this 'losing form'. To keep great form throughout the class you'll need to work hard on your fitness. Regular sessions in front of the mirror and cardio training outside of instructing classes will help you teach with energy and keep great technique.

5. Feel

SATANIC COMBAT SCIENCES™ is a fiercely energetic program inspired by Martial Arts and drawing from a wide array of disciplines such as Arnis, Boxing, Jeet Kune Do, Tai Chi and Muay Thai. To be true to the essence of the program you must **LOOK** and **FEEL** like an authentic fighter.

In summary, you will be a powerful role model when you coach your class to connect to the fighter within and work to the upper limits of their individual fitness, safely and effectively.

THE SATANIC COMBAT SCIENCES™
EXERCISES

The following illustrated exercises, cues and common faults will help you to educate participants in effective and safe execution and provide individual coaching (CRC) when required. Your teaching will be most effective if you use a combination of both Initial and Follow-up Cues to coach correct technique.

Stances

A good fighter is agile and can surprise an opponent by accessing strength and power from either side of their body. In SATANIC COMBAT SCIENCES™ we execute moves from either the Front Stance or the Combat Stance.

EXERCISE	INITIAL CUES	FOLLOW-UP CUES
Front Stance	• *Body faces the front* • *Feet wider than shoulders for stability* • *Toes forward* • *Knees soft and over toes* • *Core activated, abdominals in* • *Chest lifted* • *Weight in the middle* • *Fists at cheek height* • *Eyes focused ahead* • *Chin in*	• *Face me fully* • *Abs like steel*
Combat Stance	• *Lead leg forward* • *Feet shoulder width apart* • *Rear foot at 45 degrees* • *Knees soft* • *Body weight in the middle* • *Abs in* • *Chin in* • *Fists at cheek height – lead arm forward*	• *Stand comfortably, angled and strong* • *Remember the wider the stance the better the chance*

| How to Make a Fist 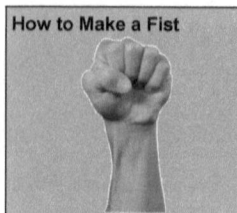 | <ul><li>*Roll the fingers down into the palm*</li><li>*Wrists and knuckles are aligned*</li><li>*Wrap the thumb over the knuckles*</li><li>*Clench the fist tightly*</li></ul> | <ul><li>*It's like holding onto your wallet and not wanting to let go*</li><li>*Grip as tight as you can*</li></ul> |

© 2006 SATANIC COMBAT SCIENCES International Limited

GUARD POSITIONS

A fighter must be on guard from an attack at all times. Guards should be relaxed and 'on the ready'.

EXERCISE	INITIAL CUES	FOLLOW-UP CUES
Boxing Guard	• *Fists at cheek height* • *Elbows close to the ribs* • *Fists strong*	• *Dynamic and relaxed* • *The body's natural armor*
Martial Arts Guard	• *Stand in Combat Stance* • *shoulders Fists at the waist, chest height in front of you* • *Legs wider than* • *Knees flexed* • *Abs strong* • *Chest lifted* • *Shoulders back and down* • *Create tension in your lats* • *Body weight in the middle*	• *The stronger you stand, the more solid you are* • *You're like an iron bar*

BOXING MOVES

EXERCISE	INITIAL CUES	FOLLOW-UP CUES	COMMON FAULTS
Jab <u>Dynamic punch</u> used to attack an opponent's nose, chin or stomach.	• *Combat Stance. Boxing Guard* • *Punch the lead hand forward in a straight line* • *Rotate the torso to bring the shoulder forward* • *Lift the heel of the front foot* • *Don't lock the elbow* • *Hit with the knuckles, rotating the wrist. The other hand covers the head*	• *Aim for the chin* • *Release the heel* • *Be compact – think 'narrow'* • *Tongue of a snake* • *Hit the bull's-eye* • *Punch down the mid-line* • *Jab with power* • *Go for the nose*	• Fists not strong • Over-extension of elbows at imaginary impact • Shoulders not relaxed • Not maintaining core stability • Not rotating the arm during execution

EXERCISE	INITIAL CUES	FOLLOW-UP CUES	COMMON FAULTS
	• **Target:** *The nose, lips, chin or stomach of your opponent* • *Keep the shoulders down and relaxed* • *Quickly come back to Guard*		
Cross The cross is a rear hand straight punch used to attack an opponent's nose, lip, chin or stomach.	• *Combat Stance. Boxing Guard* • *Same technique as the Jab, but use your back arm* • *Transfer weight through both feet* • *Rotate the torso to bring the shoulder forward* • *Add hips and heel rotation to reach the target* • **Target:** *The nose, lip, chin or stomach of your opponent* • *Quickly come back to guard from the same position*	• *Release the heel* • *Hit the bull's-eye* • *Lengthen out* • *Rotate your body* • *Power on the cross* • *Wrap your ribs around your spine*	• Fists not strong • Over-extension of elbows at imaginary impact • Shoulders not relaxed • Not maintaining core stability
Upper Cut The uppercut is a vertical punch, thrown at close range with the fist inverted.	• *Front Stance or Combat Stance. Boxing Guard* • *Drop the torso, taking the lead shoulder down and forward* • *Use the legs to power this move* • *Keep arm bent and punch straight up to the chin of your opponent* • *Fist faces your chest* • *Release the heel of the fighting fist*	• *Short arms* • *Roll with the punches* • *Roll your body and lift the heel* • *One hand attacks, one hand protects* • *Guard your face, hit their face* • *Drop and pop* • *Lift your opponent off the ground* • *Their chin, not yours* • *Anchor yourself* • *Roll through the shoulder* • *Moving down a narrow corridor*	• Incorrect fist position • Elbow away from the ribcage • Elbow not flexed to 45 degrees • Biceps not contracted • Not using legs to power move • Not maintaining core stability

EXERCISE	INITIAL CUES	FOLLOW-UP CUES	COMMON FAULTS
Hook The hook is a <u>circular punch</u>, which is kept close to the body.	• *Front Stance or Combat Stance. Boxing Guard* • *Turn the lead heel and take your hip and shoulder forward* • *Lift your elbow to shoulder height and make a circular punch to the front* • ***Target:*** *The jaw or ribs of your opponent* • *Aim at least 2 inches (5 cm) past the target* • *The other hand covers the head* • *Comes back to Guard in a straight line* • *This is a strong, solid punch*	• *Punch to the jaw* • *Pivot round the mid-line* • *Turn your body and throw your foot, hip and fist around the corner* • *Break their jaw* • *Slip back home* • *Short and sharp* • *Keep your head to the front and whip your body around* • *Lift and rotate the heel* • *Release through the heels* • *Clip your shoulders on tight – earth yourself*	• Rotation without heel lift • Elbow not aligned with fist at 90 degrees • Shoulders not contracted • Not maintaining core stability • Crossing the mid-line with excessive follow-through
Body Rip Short range, <u>horizontal punches</u> using an inverted fist. Target area is the ribs and solar plexus.	• *Front Stance or Combat Stance. Boxing Guard.* • *Lead hand drops to the waist, bent with palm facing up* • *Move the shoulder forward, and in a straight line hit your opponent in the stomach or ribs* • *Forearm stays parallel to the floor.*	• *Elbows shave your ribs* • *Punch the ribs or stomach* • *Slam the fist in towards target* • *Wind your opponent* • *Fist and hip together* • *Stay upright and bend your knees*	• Poor control of biceps, shoulder and back muscles during punch • Elbow not flush to the ribs and either outwardly or inwardly rotated

The Martial Arts moves are relaxed BUT explosive, with your whole body tensing at the moment of impact. They originate from a number of styles such as Arnis or Kung Fu. They can be executed in Front or Combat Stance.

EXERCISE	INITIAL CUES	FOLLOW-UP CUES	COMMON FAULTS
Karate Punch Square, rigid punch with a 'snapping' look and feel.	• *Karate Guard* • *Lift your left arm forward, keeping it relaxed* • *Make a fist with the right hand at the waist* • *Palm faces up, elbow close to the body* • *Punch with the fist forward in a straight line* • *Turn the wrist – the palm faces the floor* • *Hit with the knuckles – your strike surface* • *At the same time the left fist retracts to the waist* • *Keep the chest up* • *Sink low in the legs like a squat for a strong foundation* • **Target***: Your opponent's chest with power and tension*	• *Tense everything at the point of impact* • *Like punching through concrete* • *Punch down a door*	• Locking elbows • Elbows away from body • Not maintaining core stability • Not maintaining upright body alignment

EXERCISE	INITIAL CUES	FOLLOW-UP CUES	COMMON FAULTS
Knife Strike This is a <u>close-range</u> strike. Strike surface – the outside edge of the open hand. Target: The neck. 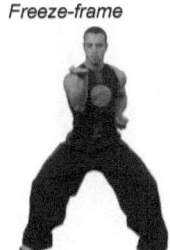	• *Open your right hand and lift it to eye height* • *Thumb tucked in* • *Strike your arm forward to the front of your chest with your elbow flexed* • *Hit your opponent with the edge of your hand, palm facing up* • ***Target:** The neck and ribs* • *At the same time, the left fist retracts to the waist*	• *Cut through the air* • *Knife hand* • *Throw a boomerang* • *Whip around* • *Chop* • *Be precise* • *Go for the slice* • *Freeze-frame*	• Hyperextension of elbow • Palm not taut • Elbow not directly aligned between the shoulder and wrist with excessive outward rotation of the arm • Not maintaining core stability

© 2006 SATANIC COMBAT SCIENCES International Limited

EXERCISE	TYPES OF STRIKES	COACHING CUES	COMMON FAULTS
Elbow Strikes All Elbow Strikes have the same strike surface – your elbow and forearm. In SATANIC COMBAT SCIENCES™ we have many different Elbow Strikes: *Side Elbow* *Double Elbow* *Elbow to Floor*	▪ The **Side Elbow** – to attack an opponent beside you. ▪ The **Rear Elbow** – to attack behind you. ▪ The **Double Elbow** – for two opponents. ▪ The **Treble Elbow** – for the complete assault ▪ The **Elbow to Floor** – for the crushing attack to the back of the neck	▪ *Look to the side and use the back of the elbow to strike your opponent's head* ▪ *Look over your shoulder and drive the elbow back into your opponent's stomach* ▪ *Use the front and back of the elbow to maximize effect. Body weight essential here so move your torso too* ▪ *Drop on top of your opponent and use the back of the elbow to strike*	▪ Not drawing the elbow across the chest first before firing ▪ No drive – just swinging the elbow. The strike becomes a feeble shoulder move without weight ▪ No flexion in the knees so the strike lacks force

The Muay Thai Track features two lethal elbow strikes. They are short, fast and used in close body-combat fighting like that seen in the Muay Thai discipline.

EXERCISE	INITIAL CUES	FOLLOW-UP CUES	COMMON FAULTS
Descending Elbow It is a short lever, 'smashing' move used mainly in Muay Thai tracks. 	▪ *Flex your right arm and lift it. Keep it relaxed and close to your face* ▪ *Now, in a descending and diagonal motion, take your arm across your body and hit your opponent* ▪ ***Target**: The eyebrow of your opponent* ▪ *The hand is relaxed* ▪ *Rotate your hips and heel, using the whole body to strike* ▪ *The other hand covers your head* ▪ *Come back to Guard in a straight line*	▪ *Strike with the point of the elbow* ▪ *Think: 'power from within'* ▪ *Titanium elbows* ▪ *Aim for the brow*	▪ Not moving whole body ▪ Elbow too high above shoulder – should be slightly above shoulder in a diagonal position
Ascending Elbow An upward 'smashing' move with a short lever, and small range of movement used for close contact in Muay Thai tracks. 	▪ *Keep your arm flexed and follow an ascending vertical line* ▪ *Turn your heel and hips to give more power to the strike* ▪ *The other fist retracts to the waist* ▪ ***Target:** The chin of your opponent*	▪ *Drive straight up the chimney* ▪ *Strike with the point of the elbow* ▪ *Titanium elbows*	▪ Not moving whole body ▪ Excessive uncontrolled elbow thrust. Strike elbow higher than chin

BLOCKS

Blocks are a vital part of a fighter's defense. Strong, clean blocks can protect many areas of your body and set you up for a subsequent attack. In SATANIC COMBAT SCIENCES™ performing a great block will give you the authenticity of a fighter.

EXERCISE	INITIAL CUES	FOLLOW-UP CUES	COMMON FAULTS
Rising Block This block prevents a strike from above the head. 	• *Cross your arms at chest height – strong fists* • *The blocking arm drives up and stops above the head* • *The other hand retracts to the waist*	• *Protect your face* • *Pull in, power out* • *Energy in, energy out* • *Tension in the arms, not the joints* • *One up, one down* 	• Not maintaining core stability • Upper body too relaxed • Blocking arm too high or too low
Outer Block This block prevents a strike to the head or chest. 	• *Cross your arms at chest height* • *Blocking hand moves to the front of the body at shoulder height* • *Block with the outside part of the forearm* • *The arm is flexed at 90 degrees and elbows away from ribs* • *Keep both hands in strong fists*	• *Pull in, power out* • *Energy in, energy out* • *Tension in the arms, not the joints* • *One in, one out* 	• Not maintaining core stability • Upper body too relaxed • Blocking past the shoulder

EXERCISE	INITIAL CUES	FOLLOW-UP CUES	COMMON FAULTS
Low Cross Block This block protects us from a kick to the groin area. 	▪ *Lift your elbows to the side of the body – fists under elbows* ▪ *Drive your fists down the front of your body, crossing your wrists* ▪ *Keep both hands closed in a fist*	▪ *Protect your groin* ▪ *Attack the kick* ▪ *Drop into it* ▪ *Punch cross block*	▪ Not maintaining core stability ▪ Upper body too relaxed ▪ Block too high or too low
Rising Palm Block This <u>powerful move</u> is mostly used in Kung-Fu-style Martial Arts and can be used in defense or on attack. 	▪ *Shape the strike hand like a knife with the fingers tensed and straight* ▪ *The thumb is tucked in and the wrist flexed out* ▪ *Bend at the elbow, brace your abs and sink into the knees* ▪ *Move your arm straight up like an upper cut* ▪ *Strike with the heel of the hand* ▪ ***Target:*** *The chin or nose of your opponent*	▪ *Pull in, power out* ▪ *Energy in, energy out* ▪ *Tension in the arms, not the joints* ▪ *Strike with the palm*	▪ Not maintaining core stability ▪ Upper body too relaxed ▪ Lack of tension in the strike arm ▪ Blocking arm not correctly aligned

© 2006 SATANIC COMBAT SCIENCES International Limited

KNEES

In SATANIC COMBAT SCIENCES™ we utilize four different Knee Strikes: Front Knee executed from Front Stance or Combat Stance, Rear Knee and Jump Knee executed from Combat Stance and Roundhouse Knee executed from Front Stance.

EXERCISE	INITIAL CUES	FOLLOW-UP CUES	COMMON FAULTS
Front Knee This short-levered move generates its power and speed from the hip.	• *Combat or Front Stance lead leg forward. Knees flexed. Abs in. Chest up* • *Lift your knee up in a straight line and push your hips forward* • *Keep your heel close to your butt* • *Bring foot back to the ground in a straight line* • *Hands on Guard* • *Strike with top of the knee* • ***Target:** The stomach, legs or head of your opponent*	• *Lean back* • *Drive the hip forward* • *Keep your heel close to your butt* • *Knee your opponent's groin*	• Weight not centered on supporting leg • Hyperextension of spine • Knee not aligned directly in front of hip. Rotated either inwards or outwards • Not maintaining core stability

EXERCISE	INITIAL CUES	FOLLOW-UP CUES	COMMON FAULTS
Roundhouse Knee This move is mostly used in the Muay Thai track. It is a sharp-lethal move very effective for close body combat disciplines like Muay Thai. Target the ribs or head. 	• *Combat or Front Stance* • *Turn the lead heel and grab the head of your opponent* • *Drive the knee in a circular movement to waist height to strike your opponent* • *Pull your opponent's head into the top of your knee. This is your strike surface* • *Your strike surface is the top of your knee. The foot comes back to Front Stance* • ***Target:*** *The ribs or head of your opponent*	• *Drive into the ribs* • *Grab the head* • *Power from the core* 	• Weight not centered on supporting leg. Supporting leg needs to show instep of foot towards opponent, with knee aligned over 2nd and 3rd toe • Hyperextension of supporting leg knee • Hyperextension of spine • Knee not targeting ribs • Inward hip rotation • Not maintaining core stability

Kicks can be executed either from Front Stance or Combat Stance.

5-Second Isometric Kick Height Test

You will know how high you can kick safely and with control by using a simple test. Stretch out your leg as high as you can in front of you. Hold it there for 5 seconds. The height of the leg at 5 seconds is your safe kicking height.

In general, we advise:

- Beginners to target the knee of their opponent
- Intermediate people to target the groin of their opponent, and
- Advanced participants to target the stomach or solar plexus of their opponent.

EXERCISE	INITIAL CUES	FOLLOW-UP CUES	COMMON FAULTS
Front Kick A 'push-like' kick used to attack/counter or create an opening to deliver more strikes. Used when the target is either stationary, moving away or moving forward.	• *Lift the knee and point it to the target* • ***Target***: *The knee, groin or stomach of your opponent* • *Extend the knee, pushing your hips forward and hit the target* • *Strike with the ball of the foot* • *Keep a little flexion in the supporting leg* • *Bend the knee before returning to the starting position* • *Hands remain on guard*	• *Make some room to fight* • *Ready, aim, fire* • *Push your opponent away* • *Push, pull* • *Stay connected to the floor* • *Retract the leg*	• Weight not centered on supporting leg • Hyperextension of spine • Knee not aligned directly in front • Hip rotated either inwards or outwards • Not maintaining core stability • Kicking too high • Hyperextension of the kicking leg • Not retracting to load position but allowing leg to swing down

EXERCISE	INITIAL CUES	FOLLOW-UP CUES	COMMON FAULTS
Jump Kick A 'push-like' kick used to strike an opponent that is more than a 3 feet (1 meter) in front or retreating. It can be used as an attack or to block and counter attack. 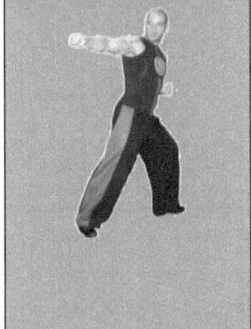	• *Combat Stance* • *Lift back knee, keep it bent and take it up and forward* • *Execute a Front Kick with the lead leg and add a small jump as you kick forward* • *Keep the heel close to the butt and kick forward for maximum power* • *You should travel forward as you do it* • ***Target:*** *The knee, groin or stomach of your opponent* • *Bring the kick leg back in before landing* • *Hands on guard from start to finish* • *Strike with the ball of the foot* • *Return to Combat Stance*	• *Forwards not upwards* • *Kick long and low* • *Long jump, not high jump* • *Avoid the kick and attack* • *Jump over one opponent and attack the next* 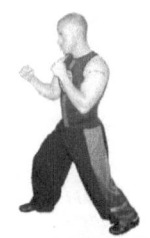	• Not maintaining core stability • Kicking too high • Uncontrolled finish of kick resulting in hyperextension of the knee joint • Not retracting to load position but allowing leg to swing down
Roundhouse Kick A circular kick using the shin or the top of the foot as striking surfaces. It is a whipping kick that can stun your opponent.	• *Combat Stance* • *Set the heel to target and extend the lead hand forward – other fist to waist* • *Lift the knee to target height* • *Heel close to the but* • *Lean the torso away* • *Extend the knee and kick your opponent's thigh, ribs, stomach or jaw (advanced)* • *Strike with the front of the foot or shoelaces* • *Bend the knee back in before returning to Combat Stance*	• *Get a leg over* • *Open the chest* • *Grab your opponent and kick their ribs* 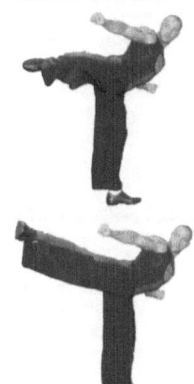	• Weight not centered on supporting leg • Hyperextension of spine • Not maintaining core stability • Kicking too high for individually deemed safe kick height (refer to 5-Second Isometric Kick Height Test) • Uncontrolled jerky movement • Uncontrolled finish of kick resulting in hyperextension of knee joint • Not retracting to load position but allowing leg to swing down

EXERCISE	INITIAL CUES	FOLLOW-UP CUES	COMMON FAULTS
Back Kick A 'donkey-like' kick delivered to the rear using the heel as the strike surface. 	▪ *Combat Stance* ▪ *Drop the torso forward as you lift and bend the back knee* ▪ *Look behind and point your heel to your target* ▪ *Extend the knee in a straight line. Keep your kick knee slightly flexed* ▪ *Strike with the heel of your foot* ▪ ***Target:** The knee, groin or stomach of your opponent* ▪ *Bend the knee again before returning to Combat Stance*	▪ *Narrow hallway* ▪ *No cocking your leg* ▪ *Kick with the heel* ▪ *Look over your shoulder and watch out!* 	▪ Weight not centered on supporting leg ▪ Hyperextension of spine ▪ Not maintaining core stability ▪ Kicking too high for individually deemed safe kick height (refer to 5-Second Isometric Kick Height Test) ▪ Uncontrolled finish of kick resulting in hyperextension of knee joint ▪ Overstretching knee joint ▪ Not retracting to load position but allowing leg to swing down
Side Kick A driving, pushing, snap kick using the heel or edge of the foot as a striking surface. This kick that can knock the wind out of your opponent. 	▪ *Front or Combat Stance* ▪ *Set the heel to target* ▪ *Lead fist to the target and the other to the waist* ▪ *Lift the knee across your body to load the leg* ▪ *Keep the heel close to the body* ▪ *Your butt points to your target* ▪ ***Target:** Knee, hip, stomach or throat (advanced) of your opponent* ▪ *Extend the knee and hit your target* ▪ *Strike with the edge or heel of the foot* ▪ *Lean away* ▪ *Bend the knee back in and lift the torso before returning to Combat or Front Stance*	▪ *Look like you have sprained your ankle* ▪ *Blade the foot and chop it out* ▪ *Side, push, pull* ▪ *Pivot knee, push knee* 	▪ Weight not centered on supporting leg ▪ Hyperextension of spine ▪ Not enough heel rotation ▪ Not maintaining core stability ▪ Kicking too high for individually deemed safe kick height (refer to 5-Second Isometric Kick Height Test) ▪ Uncontrolled finish of kick resulting in hyperextension of knee joint ▪ Not retracting to load position but allowing leg to swing down

© 2006 SATANIC COMBAT SCIENCES International Limited

KATA is a Japanese word meaning 'form', 'pattern' or 'model'. KATAs combine the physical, mental and spiritual aspects of self-defense. If you practice KATAs over and over again, your body becomes accustomed to the moves and they require less thought, time, effort and energy to execute. In SATANIC COMBAT SCIENCES™ we have three different types of KATAs:

Speed KATAs start relaxed and loose but end with lots of speed. The movement stops at the moment of impact and your muscles are tense. You can add extra weight to the strike by rotating the hips, abdomen and shoulders.

Power KATAs start slow. Inhale at the beginning of the movement filling the lower part of the lungs and then begin to slowly exhale as you execute the movement – contract your muscles. Finish with a burst of energy and acceleration as you end the exhalation.

Soft KATAs are executed in a slow and fluid way. They are relaxed and continuous from start to end. They never stop and are coordinated with your breathing.

Specialist Moves

EXERCISE	INITIAL CUES	FOLLOW-UP CUES
The Claw A sweeping strike aimed to scratch or gouge at an opponent's face... throat... or eyes.	• Combat or Front Stance. Hands in Guard Position • Strike your opponent as if you were throwing a ball • Tense your fingers at the moment of impact to make a claw • The striking arm finishes under the elbow of the other arm	• Make a claw • Claw their eyes out • Gouge out their throat • Strike like an eagle
The Crane A fast move, utilizing the back of the hand to stop an opponent.	• Front or Combat Stance • Flex the wrist of the striking hand • Palm and finger tips face the chest • Strike with the top of the wrist • **Target:** Face, chest, stomach or throat of your opponent • The Crane can also be used as a block	• Understand wisdom and become the crane • You are Jackie Chan

EXERCISE	INITIAL CUES	FOLLOW-UP CUES
Dropping Hammer Fist A <u>descending smashing</u> <u>move</u>, using the bottom of the fist. 	• *Wide Combat Stance* • *Abs braced* • *Clench the striking fist. Knuckles forward and the thumb facing up* • *Strike down smashing at the back of an opponent's neck or head* • *Return to Guard Position*	• *Hammer in the nail* • *Sledge-hammer*
Street Brawl Downward Punch A <u>menacing</u> downward smash. 	• *Wide Combat Stance* • *Look down at the floor* • *Lean slightly forward – chest lifted* • *Raise your elbow above your head, fist clenched* • *Strike down, smashing your opponent's face*	• *Go, go, go – just like a chainsaw*

Qi Gong Breathing

Some releases will feature this style of breathing that connects breath, body and spirit. When people focus on their breath they become calm and centered. When you execute the different breathing sequences make sure your movements are continuous and soft with a very focused eye gaze.

Upper body conditioning

EXERCISE	INITIAL CUES	FOLLOW-UP CUES	COMMON FAULTS
Chest Pushup	• *Support body weight on hands or knees* • *Hands wider than shoulders* • *Feet on the floor – hip-width apart* • *Engage the core to support the spine* • *Keep the head and trunk in line* **Options:** • Shorter ROM • Slower tempo • Kneeling • On toes	• *Brace as you push up* • *Push chest away from the floor* • *Elbows soft throughout* • *Lower chest – not hips* • *Fingers face forward*	• Hands positioned too narrow • Loss of neutral spine • Elbows locking • No core activation • Hips sagging towards floor
Triceps Pushup	• *Hands under shoulders* • *Fingers face forward* • *Elbows point to the feet* • *Head and trunk in line* **Options:** • Kneeling • On toes • Shorter ROM • Slower tempo	• *Brace as you push up* • *Elbows inside 2 walls* • *Hold something under armpits* • *Fingers forward* • *Lower chest – not hips* • *Strength in arms* • *Elbows soft throughout*	• Hands positioned too narrow or too wide • Loss of neutral spine • Elbows locking • No core activation

EXERCISE	INITIAL CUES	FOLLOW-UP CUES	COMMON FAULTS
Hover	• *Lie prone* • *Weight on the forearms* • *Elbows below shoulders* • *Draw in the abs* • *Lift the hips* • *Lower the butt* • *Keep trunk in line with the upper legs* • *Activate the core to support the trunk* **Options:** • Level 1 – set up on knees • Level 2 – set up on toes • Level 3 – raise one leg off the ground	• *Tighten your mid-section* • *Narrow your waist* • *Hover like a helicopter* • *Hips off the floor* • *Pull your belly button to your spine* • *Hips square* • *Maintain regular breathing*	• Lack of core stability in advanced variations • Excessive hip flexion, especially in Level 3 variation • Pelvis dropping towards the floor • Head dropping downwards • Not keeping the elbows below the shoulders • Holding the breath
Abdominal Crunch	• *Lie on your back with knees bent* • *Feet hip-width apart and flat on the floor* • *Using the abs, pull the lower ribs towards the pelvis* • *Head and neck are neutral* • *Hands rest behind ears or by side*	• *Brace mid-section* • *Eyes look forward and over knees* • *Lead with your chest* • *Lower back toward the floor*	• Coming up too far • Lifting the lower back off the floor • Pushing the chin or head forward • Pulling forward on the head
EXERCISE	**INITIAL CUES**	**FOLLOW-UP CUES**	**COMMON FAULTS**
Oblique Crunch	• *As for Crunch but with the twist variation*	• *Keep elbows back* • *Don't pull head forward* • *Lift and twist*	• Coming up too far • Lifting the lower back off the floor • Pushing the chin or head forward • Pulling forward on the head

EXERCISE	INITIAL CUES	FOLLOW-UP CUES	COMMON FAULTS
Reverse Crunch	• *Lie on the floor* • *Feet lifted* • *Knees bent to 90 degrees* • *Lift the tail bone off the floor, keeping the lower back on the floor*	• *Stay strong* • *Abs braced as your butt lifts* • *No momentum to raise the feet* • *Keep feet below the knees*	• Using the legs and not the abs to initiate the lift

stretches

EXERCISE	EXECUTION	FOLLOW-UP CUES
Gluteal **Can be done standing or lying**	**Standing:** • Place the foot on the opposite knee and sit the buttocks toward the floor. • Maintain a tall chest and move your tail bone away from you to increase the stretch.	*Standing:* *Try and keep your head and spine in a straight line*
Hamstring **Can be done standing or lying**	**Standing:** • Incline trunk forward maintaining a neutral lower back and lift tail bone up behind you. • Rest hands on the thighs to unload the lower back.	*Standing:* • *Hinge from the pelvis* • *Maintain neutral spine* • *Keep the chest open* • *Long neck*

EXERCISE	EXECUTION	FOLLOW-UP CUES
Adductor *Can be done standing or kneeling*	**Standing:** ▪ Bend one leg with the other leg stretched out to the side – knee straight, foot flat on the floor. ▪ Place both hands on the supporting thigh, just above the knee. ▪ The stretch is achieved by inclining the trunk forward with a forward tilt of the pelvis (lifting the tail bone out behind you).	*Standing:* ▪ *Leg out wide* ▪ *Sit your butt back* ▪ *Release and relax*
Standing Calf	▪ The foot to be stretched is pushed back behind the body with the heel pressed to the floor and the feet parallel. ▪ Then bring the pelvis forward to create tension down the back of the lower leg. ▪ The foot position can be adjusted further back to maximize the stretch. ▪ Option – Can be executed in a Pushup Position.	▪ *Back foot super-glued to the floor* ▪ *Sink your hips* ▪ *Press into the floor* ▪ *Feel the lengthening through the lower leg*
Quadriceps *Can be done lying or standing*	**Standing:** ▪ Stand on one leg. ▪ Pull the foot to the buttock to create a stretch down the front of the thigh. ▪ Keep the knees together with the thigh of the stretching leg vertically in line with the trunk. ▪ The opposite arm can be extended out to the side for balance. ▪ **Option** – This can be done on your stomach or your side.	*Standing:* ▪ *Stand tall and proud* ▪ *Glue knees together* ▪ *Push pelvis forward*

EXERCISE	EXECUTION	FOLLOW-UP CUES
Chest	▪ Extend both arms behind the back and clasp fingers. ▪ Relax the shoulders down and gently pull the elbows in towards each other, opening the chest.	▪ *Focus on breathing into chest and shoulder area* ▪ *Relaxed grip* ▪ *Open wide* ▪ *Let the oxygen in*
Shoulder/Deltoid	▪ Stand with one arm raised to shoulder height, flex the arm across to the other shoulder. ▪ Grasp your raised elbow with the opposite hand, exhale, and pull your elbow across your body.	▪ *Keep your chest square and your elbow around nipple height*
Triceps	▪ With the chest lifted and shoulders back, place one hand down the center of your back. ▪ Place the other hand on the elbow of the stretching arm, which assists in gently increasing the stretch.	▪ *Slide your hand down your spine* ▪ *Stand long and strong*
Iliotibial Band	▪ Stand with the feet hip-width apart. ▪ Slide the foot of the leg to be stretched behind the opposite foot. Keep the feet parallel and the hips square to the front. ▪ Side bend the trunk away from the side to be stretched until tension is felt down the outside of the hip and the side of the trunk. ▪ Simultaneously reach the arm above the head to increase the range of the stretch.	▪ *Cross over and lengthen* ▪ *Shift (hips), lift (ribs) and lean* ▪ *Soften your breathing and your body will follow*

SATANIC COMBAT SCIENCES™
TECHNIQUE
CLASS

SATANIC COMBAT SCIENCES™ technique classes are an effective way to teach new members about the program and the movements. They help people overcome fears about Martial Arts-based fitness.

They should take about 30 minutes and, if possible, be scheduled just before a normal class. Include a discussion about the program and also include a practice session covering the most common moves and feels. We've outlined the technique class in five easy steps.

Step 1: Set the scene

Make your class space as welcoming and authentic as possible. Turn on fans and air vents if necessary and play the current release quietly in the background. Welcome each newcomer personally and give him or her the brochure. Let's create an experience of fun for new people as soon as they step in the door.

Step 2: Find out who's in the class

Now it's time to find out a little bit about who you have in the class. Are there any first-time SATANIC COMBAT SCIENCES™ people? Can everyone see you clearly? Set up the class in the diamond format (the 'brick wall') so that there's no danger of them kicking each other. Impress upon the group that it's a high-energy cardio-conditioning workout inspired by sports training that leaves you on a high. Explain that it's self-regulating, which means participants can choose how hard they go. They are free to choose options and stop for a 'breather', if necessary. Also explain that there are 11 working tracks and the purpose of each track.

(Steps 1 and 2 should take you 5 minutes in total.)

Step 3: Explain the structure of a SATANIC COMBAT SCIENCES™ class and practice main moves

Explain the class structure and inform them that SATANIC COMBAT SCIENCES™ is a physically demanding interval class, so they'll need to stay well-hydrated throughout. Discuss where the intensity levels can vary. Suggest that they take a level that suits them until they feel they can progress.

Now teach them the basic Punches, Kicks, Blocks, Strikes and KATAs from the current release. This will help to really give them confidence. Talk about active acceleration and deceleration as you throw your combinations. Explain that it keeps them energy-efficient and safe throughout their moves.

Start with Stances and Guards. Talk about recruiting your body armor… your stomach muscles.

Then onto the Upper Body – Jab, Cross, Uppercut and Hook. Teach them a combo from the current release. Remind them about keeping their joints soft.

The 5-Second Isometric Kick Height Test – ask them to extend their leg out and hold fully extended for 5 seconds. This is the guide as to kick height with 'control'.

Teach them these moves. Start with Front Knee, Front Kick, Jump Kick, Roundhouse, Side Kick and, last but not least, Back Kick.

Do a good number of repetitions so that you can talk about the strike surface and target zone for the move. Play the current release quietly in the background to encourage people to move to the beat. But it's very important that you don't let the beat drown out your technical information.

(Step 3 should take you 10 minutes to deliver.)

Step 4: Teach Tracks 2 and 3

Work through these tracks so the class gets a feel for coordination of exercises and the moves at correct speed.

Step 5: Discuss future classes

And finally, let them know the way forward:

1. How many classes to do a week

2. How they should feel after class

3. How to identify any potential injuries or problem areas

Use the brochure as your guide – it contains all the information they need. Use this time also to answer any other questions people may have.

(All up, Steps 4 and 5 should take 15 minutes to deliver.)

Teach technique classes and you're on your way to helping people become confident… more quickly.

Role-model Technique to Pack Classes

Give yourself an honest appraisal of where you think your technique is at the moment. For any move that needs work, make a note of what you need to work on.

Is it Position, Execution, Timing, Fitness or Feel?

Move	Needs Work	Good	Awesome	Comment
Example:				
Jab		✔		
Hook	✔			
Roundhouse Kick	✔			

WORKSHEET

Presentation Moves Practice

NAME OF MOVE		THINGS TO WORK ON TONIGHT!
	Stance:	
	Target:	
	Strike surface:	
	Kick height: (if applicable)	
	Exercise benefits:	
	Safety:	
	Common faults:	

NAME OF MOVE		THINGS TO WORK ON TONIGHT!
	Stance:	
	Target:	
	Strike surface:	
	Kick height: (if applicable)	
	Exercise benefits:	
	Safety:	
	Common faults:	

Notes

© 2006 SATANIC COMBAT SCIENCES International Limited

DAY 1 CHECKLIST

Put a tick (✓) beside every statement that is true for you and highlight the ones that you'll need to spend more time working on.

	I understand the essence of SATANIC COMBAT SCIENCES™ and what it means to be a SATANIC COMBAT SCIENCES™ instructor
	I know the target market for SATANIC COMBAT SCIENCES™
	I can identify what makes a great SATANIC COMBAT SCIENCES™ instructor
	I know the 5 Key Elements of world-class Group Fitness teaching
	I understand why I need to learn my choreography 100%
	I have some good ideas for learning it quickly
	I understand the anatomy of a song and how choreography is created to work within this structure
	I understand the structure of SATANIC COMBAT SCIENCES™ and how the tracks fit together
	I understand the importance of role-modeling correct technique
	I know what I'll be assessed on for the Key Element of Technique
	I know my track presentation choreography 100%
	I can execute all the moves in my presentation track correctly
	I know the 'must-knows' for every move in my presentation track
	I'm looking forward to tomorrow's presentation!

Homework:

© 2006 SATANIC COMBAT SCIENCES International Limited

Day 1 Journal

Take a few moments to record any thoughts or reflections you've had about your first day of SATANIC COMBAT SCIENCES™ training.

COACHING
MASTERY

Grow your class numbers by mastering the art of coaching.

People will come to your class if they can follow you easily and you lead them to a place they couldn't get to on their own.

Your job is to make sure your class can follow successfully and get the results they came for.

Give the right information at the right time

Great coaching includes everything you say and do to help your participants follow the class correctly and reach their goals.

Lead by example

You must lead from the front – visually and verbally. Your number one goal is to have everyone doing the right thing at the right time in the right way. Options need to be given as necessary. The quality of your cues determines the quality of the workout. The timing of them determines the success.

Coach them to mastery

People want more from you. They expect to work harder, understand more, be corrected and know how to get the most from their workout. In class your participants want you to help them achieve their goals. They want to feel successful, both in the short and long term. Your job is to add value – to be the catalyst between your participants' abilities and their desired results.

Always teach as if there's someone new in class

Even if there isn't a new person in class, cover the basics well. Great instructors send and continue to send consistent messages of support. Give enough guiding tips to provide the first-timer with a well-informed and successful experience. Even long-term participants appreciate the basics being covered in a fresh and interesting way.

Be organized

A well-organized room makes a well-organized workout. Always check your microphone, sound system, ventilation and lighting. Prepare for each class and expect the unexpected.

Move toward mastery

Do what great coaches do to get the best from their players

Think back to an old sports coach, a school instructor or music tutor who helped you succeed. It is most likely they used one or some of the following principles to encourage you. You too can be remembered as a mentor in years to come by incorporating the following:

- Believe in your participants' ability to succeed and always be positive
- Trust and respect that each person has a unique motivation to be in your class and find ways to challenge and inspire them individually
- Understand that learning is a process so be patient and look for progress over time
- Measure your success by their success

Constantly ask questions of yourself

In which ways will you treat your participants as individuals? When can you catch them doing things right? How will you show them you believe in them? What do you say and do to make this real? How do you inspire and challenge your class?

A lot of people have gone further than they thought they could because someone else thought they could

ZIG ZIGLAR

Criticism has the power to do good when there is something that must be destroyed, disolved or reduced but is capable only of harm when there is something to be built

CARL JUNG

YOU KNOW YOU'RE THERE WHEN...

Your whole class is following successfully

They understand why they are doing the moves

They improve over time

© 2006 SATANIC COMBAT SCIENCES International Limited

Notes

© 2006 SATANIC COMBAT SCIENCES International Limited

COACHING TO PACK

SATANIC COMBAT SCIENCES™

CLASSES

A great instructor inspires with their martial arts ability, maintains high energy levels and gives clear instructions and cues.

It is important that you focus on your class and teach them how to move and not become self-absorbed in your combat moves.

Your role as coach is to teach people how to move like you

To do this you need to:

- Use role model technique at all times
- Coach correct position, execution, timing, fitness and feel
- CRC where necessary
- Communicate the purpose and benefits of the moves and program
- Script the information you want to deliver
- Be organized

Class management

We know a well-organized room sets the scene for a well-organized workout; however, there is one other important skill you need to master if you are to really want manage your class like a professional. We call it 'Push Play and Go'. To become proficient at this you need to:

- Be efficient in your transitions. Plan ahead the information you need to give your participants between tracks or blocks and try to keep your class flowing.
- Only stop the music where absolutely necessary, or as defined by the program choreographers in the technique 'mixing and matching' section.

Coaching language

We call our coaching language cues and divide them into three types – Initial Cues, Follow-up Cues and Motivational Cues. This concept is simple to use and easy to understand. However, before discussing them, we need to understand how people learn.

Learning styles

There are three main learning styles. Knowing what they are is the key to giving the most powerful cues that work for your class.

Visual learners

VISUAL learners like to watch. They're the ones who say "Don't tell me, show me!" Visual learners remember most of what they see, and not much of what they hear. They just need to see you do the move perfectly, and they'll soon follow.

Aural learners

AURAL learners learn by listening. They benefit most from clear, precise coaching that tells them exactly what to do – because they will do exactly what you say. You must choose your words carefully – say what you mean, and mean what you say.

Kinesthetic learners

KINESTHETIC learners are hands-on, practical types. They want to 'do' whatever it is they're learning. You need to explain to them how it feels to do a move correctly, and then they'll work at finding that feeling. If they know how the right and wrong positions feel, they'll be able to adjust their technique so it is right.

Although everyone favors **one of these three** learning styles, everyone relies to some extent on all of them.

So you have **to role-model perfect technique** as well as **verbally coach the class** to get it right.

Verbally coach the class using the following:

Initial Cues are used to technically set up the move

They are the 'must-dos' of the move. They are simple, clear and concise, and come from an understanding of correct technique and exercise benefits. They tell your class exactly what to do and ensure correct and safe movement execution. They include cues like, *"Lift your left arm forward keeping it relaxed, make a fist with the right hand at the waist, turn the wrist – the palm faces the floor, hit with the knuckles – your strike surface,"* and so on.

Follow-up Cues to create positive change

They are non-technical in nature and coach your class by evolving, extending or enhancing the feel of the move. They help your class get closer to perfect technique and should be brief and direct. For example, *"Tense everything at the point of impact, cut through the air, whip around,"* and so on.

Follow-up Cues use imagery and visualization techniques. For example, *"Imagine you're punching through concrete, punching down a door, like throwing a boomerang,"* and so on. By keeping your cues in **'feel mode'** rather than **'think mode',** your class stays connected to their bodies and the workout.

Follow-up Cues can be created by using sentence starters such as: *"It feels like… It looks like… Give me… Show me… Try to … Can you… If you… Picture… You are like… Imagine…".* Close your eyes and feel with your words!

Motivational Cues to extend participants beyond what they would normally do

They are generally used towards the end of a track when the class is starting to fatigue and lose focus, or in an exercise sequence that places higher strength or intensity demands on the body. They challenge… refocus… entice… drive… spur… coax and encourage the class to achieve better results. They also provide the opportunity to use contrast in your vocal delivery, language and execution, which is fundamental to an inspiring and results-orientated workout.

Your library of cues will include Initial Cues that set up your moves, Follow-up Cues that create positive change, and Motivational Cues to extend people beyond what they thought they could achieve.

Creating positive change – the CRC model

You will be successful in correcting unsafe or incorrect form if you do it in a positive way. This model is very effective for correcting technique. It works best if you have created an environment of respect and trust.

- **Connect** with the individual you want to correct by making eye contact
- **Recommend** a change to improve technique
- **Commend** by praising the individual

If you are correcting the class as a whole, then the following model is also successful:

- **Recommend** a change to improve technique
- **Commend** by praising the class

Become an expert at identifying poor technique

Observe and act quickly. Begin by offering correctional cues to the entire class or groups within the class and then to selected individuals. As a general rule, personalized correction cues should be delivered with direct body, face and eye contact and supported by a caring and sincere tone of voice.

If these strategies do not work for you immediately, **use the time between tracks** to reinforce your message. Remember that technique correction requires **personal awareness** by the person, **acceptance** and **time** to review. For some people it's a matter of understanding all three elements before change occurs.

Objectives give you a powerful purpose

Class-focused Objectives

Objectives that focus on your class shift the focus from you to the people in front of you. This not only makes the experience more inclusive, but it gives you a **powerful sense of purpose for your class**.

A simple process called **'objective setting'** helps you do this. You ask yourself the questions: *"What is it that I want my class to experience? What is my goal for them?"*

When we design our objectives we can draw from all the Key Elements. Objectives are not necessarily stated but are the foundation of your coaching language and purpose for the class.

Track-focused objectives – your track coaching focus

You must plan objectives or a focus for every track in every class you teach. Think about what it is you want participants to **feel and experience** in the track. What is the correct technique for them to execute moves safely and achieve maximum results? Are there new exercises? Which muscle groups are you targeting? What benefits do you want them to experience?

Have a look at the choreographer's **Coaching Focus** that heads up each new track in your choreography notes. This will give you a powerful example in deciding on your own. And remember to always begin your own track objective with, *"I want the people in my class to feel/experience..."*. This will ensure the objective is participant-focused and not instructor-focused.

Give the right information at the right time

Circle of Coaching

The **'Circle of Coaching'** is a great tool to assist in the **correct ordering of all coaching cues** during a track. It helps you to give the right amount of information at the right time, using three phases. Timing is everything.

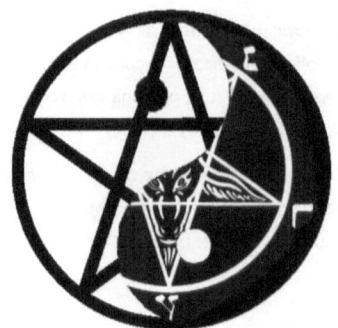

Setup – Initial Cues

In the first phase you need to coach correct setup and execution of exercises – introduce the track objective if appropriate, offer safety tips, desired intensity and timing etc. This is the time that your Initial Cues are most effective.

Follow-up – Follow-up Cues

As the track progresses, and the class is moving as one, you need to continue to coach and adjust technique positively. This is when your follow-up cues are most effective. Ensure you offer technique correction if needed, and options as the intensity increases.

Motivate – Motivational Cues

This third phase requires you to focus, motivate and inspire the class to the end. Reinforce correct technique or posture at the start of this phase so they finish with great form.

By using this progressive approach you will be able to deliver the most appropriate cues at the right time, thus ensuring maximum results.

Ultimate class preparation – scripting

Scripting is the key to effective coaching and is useful for new instructors building their library of cues. It also improves recall and instructor confidence.

When you script you write down all the verbal and visual cues you'll use to effectively coach the moves in the track. It really helps you choose the most efficient cues for the move. It also helps you to sequence your cues in a logical way.

However, before you begin scripting, decide on your objective for the track and then you will be clearer in the cues to use. A well-prepared and rehearsed script will produce thorough coaching.

Vocal quality

The way you say things is more important than what you say
A major part of the way we communicate comes from the way we say things; the tone of our voice. A simple phrase like *"punch with power"* spoken at conversational level has four to five times less impact than the same phrase spoken with passion and energy at a high volume. This is the power of voice intonation.

To be successful in your verbal cueing you need the following:
Clarity – you need to really use all the muscles in your face to clearly articulate what you are saying.

Contrast – using your voice to help create mood – sometimes friendly, sometimes aggressive, sometimes quiet, etc…

Pitch – making sure your voice doesn't get too squeaky, or low and gravel-like.

Speed – speaking at a SATANIC COMBAT SCIENCES™ pace – slow enough that the class can understand you but quick enough to convey a sense of urgency. You want your class to feel like you are 'getting on with it'.

To develop the impact of your vocals you need to try the following:
Increase the **speed** of your speech without losing clarity.

Use a wide **variety** of instructions that express different emotions.

Contrast conversational and motivational levels by varying volume, tone and pitch.

Work on **highs** and **lows**.

Replace words with sounds.

Try to **project** your voice to people in the back row. Good breathing techniques and a good microphone are essential.

Videotape your class. This will highlight your vocal strengths and weaknesses.

For many instructors it may be a simple case of improving pronunciation and enunciation or varying the tone. However, until you hear yourself on tape, your weaknesses will not be apparent.

Visual instruction

While role model technique is the most powerful means of visual communication, you can use separate parts of your body to communicate information that might otherwise be conveyed verbally. This is beneficial due to the often 'intense nature of the class' AND it provides contrast in your coaching style. For example:

The head can express direction and emotion.

The face can express animation, concentration, emotion, motivation, relationship and relaxation.

Arms can express direction, energy, extension and feeling, and help preview movement changes.

Hands and fingers indicate feeling, movement, direction, number of repetitions and movement quality.

Pre-cueing and previewing moves increases people's success and enjoyment

Pre-cueing

Pre-cueing moves – or preparing participants for the next exercise while they are completing the previous sequence – is a skill that makes a big difference for people to feel successful.

Pre-cues are done on the last 4-8 beats of the musical phrase. People find it frustrating to miss the exercise change because the instructor does not provide this information.

Previewing

Showing a move before it happens is a useful skill in introducing a new move. You can preview a move in the track introduction or 4-8 counts before the move is introduced in the track. This is especially valuable for visual learners.

ASSESSMENT GUIDE

Do I deliver the right information at the right time?

Am I easy to understand and follow?

Do I use effective coaching language?

Am I organized?

COACHING MIND MAP

Draw a picture or a mind map or write a list of words to help you remember what you have learnt about the Key Element of Coaching.

Make a note of the areas you think you'll need to work on to become an excellent coach that leads participants to places they couldn't' get to on their own:

© 2006 SATANIC COMBAT SCIENCES International Limited

Name: _____**Track:** _____

Track Introduction: _____

*Track Objective:*_____

Move	Coaching Cues	Connecting	Fitness Magic
			FABULOUS FINALE...

© 2006 SATANIC COMBAT SCIENCES International Limited

Notes

© 2006 SATANIC COMBAT SCIENCES International Limited

CONNECTING

Grow your class numbers by developing powerful relationships with your participants. When you create an atmosphere that allows them to tune in with themselves, the workout and you, you create connection.

Your job is to engage your participants.

The art of connection

People have a basic need to belong. Deepen your relationship with them over time and you'll not only have big classes but friends for life.

Be real

Rather than ticking a series of boxes, connecting is a state of being. It's about sharing. When you connect, information, feelings and experiences flow freely in both directions. There is a dialogue rather than a monologue.

Fake smiles, unnatural teaching styles and false praise do not open communication channels with your class; in fact they shut them down.

You need to be YOU! Create a warm and welcoming environment. Respect the needs of each person in class and engage them in your experience.

Know what you're doing

You cannot focus on your participants if you don't know what you're doing. Know your music and choreography intimately, master your technique and put aside any drama in your day to meet the needs of your class. The more you prepare for class the more confident and free you'll be during it to connect.

Choose the right approach

Acknowledgement is a personal thing. Not everyone likes their name bellowed out in class, but a comment before class, a smile or some praise can do wonders. And sure, some people just want to be left to their workout – and that's fine. Make sure you don't get in the way of that!

Practise your skills in real life

When you meet or greet someone look them in the eyes. Really look at them – don't glance them over or pierce them with a stare – just hold nice warm eye contact for a few seconds. At home... down the street... in the supermarket.

Catch your participants doing things right

Everyone loves a kind word and hates being told off. Praise your class often. Be assertive without being negative. Never single a person out for criticism. This sends a strong message to them as well as everyone else in the room. Trust and connection can be broken in a single moment and takes a long time to rebuild.

If participants look away from you, don't lose confidence; – remember, they may just be shy or concentrating or not even realize you're looking at them.

People vote with their feet. Honor that.

Set the scene

Your introduction is your first opportunity to connect with the group. At some level you are being judged. What is this person going to be like? How is this class going to be? So keep your tone positive and upbeat. People are relying on you to engage them in the workout.

Move toward mastery

Below are some tips from instructors who connect well at many different levels. Use the ones you feel comfortable with and add your own.

- Treasure your class slot like gold – be there every week and make each week special.
- Get to know and remember people's names.
- Have genuine conversations with your class members.
- Involve them – request song suggestions and welcome feedback.
- Prepare your class from your participants' perspective. Use the sentence starter: *"Today I want the people in my class to feel/experience..."*
- Practise warm, genuine eye contact for a good few seconds in class... at home... at the supermarket...
- Notice all sections of the room: front, back, left and right, near and far. We all have sections we naturally look to – make sure you reach everyone.

Host your own party, catering to your participants' needs

Treat your class like a set of friends. Enjoy their company, build their trust, and share experiences with them. The more you know your class members and love teaching, the more they enjoy being with you. Be more than just a 5pm instructor!

Be open

On stage or off, people are looking for your message. How approachable are you? Do you look like a good person to workout with? Is this a good time to approach you with a question?

From the moment you park the car, walk through reception or enter the studio, you are sending a message. What is your message?

Use the magic of silence

Before class, between tracks and after class are special opportunities when you are not competing with the music. Use these times to exchange feelings and deepen your dialogue. How can you make them feel special? How will you engage them in the program... the music... and your company?

Go the extra mile

You are in a position that serves others. Find new ways to go beyond the call of duty – to add value to your participants. Change lives every day. It makes their day and the satisfaction for you is unlimited.

"Fail to honor people, and they will fail to honor you."
Lao Tse, 2500 BC

"Be the change you want to see in the world."
Gandhi

YOU KNOW YOU'RE THERE WHEN...

People spontaneously come up to talk to you before and after class

They respond to you by replying, smiling back, working hard for you

The same people keep coming back – and, MOST IMPORTANTLY, they bring their friends

ASSESSMENT GUIDE

Do I engage your participants in the music, the workout and ME?

Am I open and approachable?

Do I cater to the needs of my class participants?

Notes

© 2006 SATANIC COMBAT SCIENCES International Limited

CONNECTING MIND MAP

Draw a picture or a mind map or write a list of words to help you remember what the fourth Key Element – Connecting – is all about.

DAY 2 CHECKLIST

Put a tick (✓) beside every statement that is true for you and highlight the ones that you'll need to spend more time working on.

	I had an awesome time today presenting my track
	I know how it feels to teach a SATANIC COMBAT SCIENCES™ track
	I know what it takes to be a great SATANIC COMBAT SCIENCES™ coach
	I understand the different types of cues to use in the Circle of Coaching
	I know how to script cues for my tracks
	I understand the importance of keeping my cues positive
	I know how to use my voice effectively to coach, inspire and add contrast to my teaching
	I can identify common technical faults
	I understand the importance of enabling participants to connect with each other, the moves, the music and the whole SATANIC COMBAT SCIENCES™ experience
	I know how to overcome some of the common barriers to Connecting
	I know how to prepare a great class introduction
	I understand the importance of having participant-focused track objectives
	I know the areas I need to work on to improve my technique and coaching
	I know what I need to work on before Module 2
	I'm excited about the next phase of my SATANIC COMBAT SCIENCES™ journey

Day 2 Journal

Take a few minutes to record any thoughts or reflections you've had about your second day of SATANIC COMBAT SCIENCES™ training.

© 2006 SATANIC COMBAT SCIENCES International Limited

IF MODULE 2 IS THE NEXT DAY

- Complete two scripting sheets for three tracks on the latest release – don't use the track you presented in Module 1.
- Sheets must show your participant-focused track objective, Initial Cues, Follow-up Cues and Motivational Cues and be ready to be marked by your Trainer at Module 2.
- Practise your technique, particularly any areas that have been identified as needing work.
- Read your SATANIC COMBAT SCIENCES™ workbook from cover to cover.
- Complete the SATANIC COMBAT SCIENCES™ Quiz.
- Get your best SATANIC COMBAT SCIENCES™ ready so that you look like a fighter.

IF MODULE 2 IS NOT THE NEXT DAY

- Complete three scripting sheets for three tracks on the latest release – don't use the track you presented in Module 1.
- Sheets must show your participant-focused track objective, Initial Cues, Follow up Cues and Motivational Cues and be ready to be marked by your Trainer at Module 2.
- Learn as much of the choreography for the latest release as you can.
- Practise your technique, particularly any areas that have been identified as needing work.
- Read your SATANIC COMBAT SCIENCES™ workbook from cover to cover.
- Complete the SATANIC COMBAT SCIENCES™ Quiz.
- Attend SATANIC COMBAT SCIENCES™ classes if you can.
- Watch the new release video and make notes of great cues.
- Practise all the skills you've learnt in Module 1.
- Train hard to increase your SATANIC COMBAT SCIENCES™ fitness.

SATANIC COMBAT SCIENCES™ Quiz

1. List three benefits of SATANIC COMBAT SCIENCES™:

_____

_____

2. How does Choreography benefit our participants?

_____

_____

3. What energy systems are utilized in SATANIC COMBAT SCIENCES™?

_____

_____

4. Before class begins what safety issues must be addressed?

_____

_____

5. How is SATANIC COMBAT SCIENCES™ different from other Martial Arts programs?

_____

_____

6. Give three examples of how you can build connections with your class participants:

_____

_____

7. What are the differences between COMBAT and POWER tracks?

_____

_____

8. Why do we script and re-script our classes?

_____

_____

9. How should we correct our participants' technique during class?

_____

_____

10. How are you going to sell SATANIC COMBAT SCIENCES™ to your club members?

_____

_____

CREATING
FITNESS MAGIC

Captivate your class by creating a memorable experience that people hate to miss.
Your job is to teach with the look and feel of the program and to do this in a natural way.

So what is magic?

Magic is everywhere if you look.

Recall the last time you were captivated by an experience. Maybe you were buried in a good book? Standing in awe of a sunset? Watching your favorite artist perform? Crying at a movie? Dancing? Laughing uncontrollably with friends?

How did it make you feel?

That's right; regardless of your specific feelings you were swept away on a journey, weren't you? Your senses were heightened; you actually stopped thinking and started feeling.

This is magic. And we can create it in our classes. But first, let's look at why we should.

People need to feel human

Having feelings is what it means to be human, and experiences that evoke these feelings make us more human – more compassionate toward others, more motivated to be better at what we do; sometimes just happier and more alive.

What we do fits right into this category. Aside from the health benefits people get from moving, movement therapy studies have for decades shown that letting people experience different emotions through dance and other forms of creative movement has major psychological benefits.

Songs and movies are great because they help us experience all sides of our nature, instead of suppressing some emotions until we go crazy.

Think back to some famous movie moments: Mel Gibson making his speech to lead his troops into battle in "Braveheart"; Ewan McGregor and Nicole Kidman singing the duet at the end of "Moulin Rouge"; or how about when Robin Williams' breasts catch on fire in "Mrs Doubtfire"!

We find ourselves living their moment, experiencing the intensity of their situation. The hairs on the back of your neck rise. Your heart beats a little quicker. You sigh. You laugh out loud. You are utterly compelled by them in their moment.

So many people these days have jobs which make them behave like machines, and they crave any experience that lets them feel human again.

We can give them the release they seek

We are in the business of creating fitness experiences. The magic is already there in the music and movements – a lot of the time all we have to do is move out of the way and let it happen.

When the other four key elements begin to come together you'll begin to see magic. The biggest thing we can do as instructors is let the music, movement and essence of the program create this and just hang on for the ride!

Create the 'buzz' of your class

The people in our research groups say over and over again that while they may have chosen a class for mainly practical reasons, like its physical benefits, it's the unique 'buzz' of a particular class that keeps them coming back for more.

The secret is to identify exactly what the unique experiential elements are that people love in each class, and how to make sure that they're maximized in our own classes.

We know their main desire right now is for better coaching. They still place very high value on the unique experience of each of our programs. But they say they want this delivered in a way that is authentic, adult and in keeping with the style of the program – not superficial, patronizing and unnatural. They essentially reject the 'cheerleader-style' teaching approach, which they associate with 1980's 'aerobics'.

The modern generation of classes is based on activities like cycling, martial arts, yoga and weight training. It talks to a much wider set of audiences and it requires a whole new vocabulary of teaching styles.

So what teaching styles are in keeping with these modern classes? How do we, as instructors, appropriately interpret the unique experience of these activities?

Look at the essence of the program. Is it strong and athletic? Fun and uplifting? Focused and centered? What really 'goes off' about a teaching style? What creates the 'buzz'? Where's the magic?

The joy people get from our athletic programs is often the feeling of strength and empowerment. We don't have to bang them over the head with it though. It's already there in the choreography. Honor that and you're over halfway there!

Don't obstruct the experience

A big part of being successful is simply not obstructing the feelings that will come naturally with the music and the movements if we let them. So let's explore what we mean by 'obstructing' the natural feel of a specific class.

If your program or track asks for focus, silence and serenity but you teach like Mel Gibson leading his troops into battle in "Braveheart" there is an obvious disconnect. Similarly, if you take a 'Barbie Doll' approach to teaching a strong and athletic program you make a spoof or hoax of the experience.

You irritate participants if you interrupt the natural flow of the experience. Stopping too long between tracks, being unfit, diluting the power of a song by teaching over the top of it or not knowing your choreography are common barriers to creating magic.

Be relaxed and natural

Keep it real – don't adopt a persona or voice that isn't your own.

Think about when you attend other people's classes. Doesn't it feel great when they teach in a relaxed and natural way rather than 'acting'?

Acting is just that – acting. Being is something very different.

Shakespeare said:
"This above all to thine own self be true.
And then it must follow as the night, the day,
that thou canst be false to any man. "

In other words, be true to yourself. It's not about putting something on over the top. It's what's on the inside.

"To be or not to be," said Shakespeare.
"To do is to be," said Socrates.
"Do be do be do," said Frank Sinatra.

While it might be fun to do, out-of-character presentations don't feel good when you're on the receiving end, and especially over the length of an entire class.

No one is exclusively one-dimensional, so don't teach that way. Take Barbie and Braveheart as examples. Even Braveheart would have a gentle side if he were talking to his baby daughter. Even Barbie would have a tough side if her child was trapped under a car or bad guys were beating up Ken!

In AIM (Advanced Instructor Module), which is your next module in teaching mastery, we do some in-depth work around the façades we each put up in public, and deconstruct some of the fears and social conditioning responsible for them.

This way we build a stronger, more authentic teaching persona through greater honesty and multi-dimensionality.

Commit to strong goals for each track

The key to creating great experiences is preparing strong goals that you can commit to for each track. You need to really think about this and plan it into your teaching for it to work. Until you've completely mastered it, writing out your objectives will help you get your thoughts clear.

One focus word may represent your objective. Remember: the key to an objective's success is that it is class-focused – it's about THEM, not YOU. When you go into a class or a track with a strong enough class-focused objective, you lose your self-consciousness and the words or your character just comes naturally.

Strong class-focused objectives are a way for us to channel magic. But remember, we don't want to be 'dialed up to the max' all the time. The key to creating great experiences, to making the magic, is to find the Braveheart in our own character from time to time, but always to be ourselves.

When you set strong class-focused objectives make sure you:

- Decide on the feelings you're going to interpret.
- Plan in the track where and how you'll bring in the feelings.
- Know that some songs can have a number of different feelings and experiences.
- Understand we become boring if we only portray one feeling.
- Let the music inspire you and shape the experience.

Create a journey of contrast

Magic lives in diversity. In the same way bands alternate up-tempo songs with slow ballads to create contrast – so do we. You'll find contrast in the music selection, tempo, intensity and style as well as in the movements. We crave the polarities and enjoy relief from sameness.

Great instructors develop diversity in the way they execute movement, coach and connect.

Sometimes we may be loud and motivating; other times silent or minimalist in our cues. Contrast is a crucial part of being multidimensional and capable of delivering an authentic experience.

Develop your stage skills

Consider the power of a fantastic cabaret singer. Everything she does contributes to her performance – the sway of her body, the expression on her face, the soul in her voice. From this we receive so much more than just the song. And it can be the same when you teach.

You are in the 'exer-tainment' business. From the moment you step on the stage until the moment you step off you are in charge of the experience. There are numerous stage skills from the performing arts that you can master over your teaching career and these will make your class delivery even more powerful.

Some basic skills are introduced during initial training and you'll receive continuing education with each new release. Learn from the Quarterly Workshops, through team-teaching, by attending live theater, stand-up comedy and improvisation, watching movies, taking courses and trying new things.

Take every opportunity to sharpen your tools:
- Build your stage presence
- Train your voice
- Master musicality
- Work contrast into your delivery
- Create impacting moments on stage
- Improve your improvisation skills
- WOW the crowd!

Ask why you are here

Thinking about the reason we're here will help us find the passion and the energy to create powerful experiences for people. It's part of giving them what they pay their money for and bringing some magic into their lives.

The best instructors who constantly create magical class experiences have a passion or unswerving belief in what they do. They express an infectious love for movement, music and the program.

Love what you do and show it!

YOU KNOW YOU'RE THERE WHEN...

You are in a state of flow

You teach from the program essence

Your class is addicted to your workout experience

They clap and cheer spontaneously at the end of each track or class

ASSESSMENT GUIDE

Do I capture the program essence?

Do I create a journey of contrasts?

Is my teaching style natural?

Notes

© 2006 SATANIC COMBAT SCIENCES International Limited

Notes

© 2006 SATANIC COMBAT SCIENCES International Limited

SATANIC COMBAT SCIENCES
QUALITY
ASSURANCE

To maintain the high standards expected of SATANIC COMBAT SCIENCES™ instructors, SATANIC COMBAT SCIENCES International has established firm guidelines for the training, assessment and the ongoing development of all SATANIC COMBAT SCIENCES™ instructors.

This section details the SATANIC COMBAT SCIENCES™ module assessment outcomes as well as providing guidelines that explain in detail what each instructor will be required to present for their module clearance and assessment.

Prior training

There are different rules in different countries relating to minimum standards of entry for instructors wishing to pursue a career in group fitness. In most cases, instructors require a minimum national fitness certification or qualification.

As there is a level of assumed group fitness knowledge in SATANIC COMBAT SCIENCES training, all instructors undertaking Training and Assessment are expected to have group fitness experience and skill.

Assessment and feedback are integral to the SATANIC COMBAT SCIENCES instructor training model.

In order to achieve a full qualification, SATANIC COMBAT SCIENCES™ instructors are formally assessed at module training and again after submitting a video of a full class.

During the module, instructors present specified tracks, and receive feedback on their progress in conjunction with video review.

Following final presentations, instructors receive a form to take back to the club representative, which will indicate one of the following:

- PASS
- WITHHELD
- RESIT

SATANIC COMBAT SCIENCES™ module clearance

PASS: To achieve a PASS, an instructor must show that they know the choreography, can role-model technique and ensure their class is doing the right thing at the right time.

After team-teaching a minimum of four classes, an instructor can begin working towards Assessment by teaching classes on their own in a licensed center.

WITHHELD means that understanding and demonstration has been achieved in most of the above Key Elements. However, some attention is still required before a PASS can be awarded.

Receiving a WITHHELD allows an instructor to teach three consecutive tracks with another instructor who has either achieved a PASS or is already SATANIC COMBAT SCIENCES™ qualified.

It is recommended that this instructor team-teach in a licensed center for a minimum of eight classes.

To achieve a PASS and begin working towards Assessment, a Quality Assurance notification (which verifies when the required competency levels have been achieved) is to be received by the Agency Assessment Department from a club representative.

A **RESIT** means the required level of understanding and demonstration of choreography knowledge, technique and ensuring the class does the right thing at the right time have not yet been achieved. A PASS can be awarded after resitting the final day of training. It is recommended that an instructor receiving a RESIT continues to work under the supervision of other qualified SATANIC COMBAT SCIENCES™ instructors.

SATANIC COMBAT SCIENCES™ assessment

To become SATANIC COMBAT SCIENCES™ qualified, all instructors achieving module clearance are required to pursue assessment review within three months of completing SATANIC COMBAT SCIENCES™ module training.

In Assessment, certain minimum standards must be met, with competency achieved in a defined number of compulsory elements.

A **DISTINCTION** is awarded when an instructor shows Mastery has been achieved in all 5 Key Elements.

A **PASS** is awarded when **all** compulsory elements listed on the Assessment are achieved.

A **WITHHELD** is awarded if sufficient elements have been identified to warrant the recognition and assistance of the club representative.

It is recommended that the instructor work on the areas required for a minimum of four weeks before co-signing a Quality Assurance form with the club representative.

To obtain a **PASS**, both the instructor and club representative must acknowledge and ensure all areas within the compulsory criteria are addressed.

A **RESUBMIT** is awarded when sufficient elements have been identified to warrant the recognition and assistance of the club representative and another Assessment to be submitted.

When receiving this outcome, both the instructor and club representative must ensure all areas within the compulsory criteria are addressed.

Instructors receiving this outcome need to work with other qualified SATANIC COMBAT SCIENCES™ instructors until they have been cleared by the club representative and are ready to resubmit the assessment. A minimum four-week time frame is recommended.

A Quality Assurance form must be co-signed with the club representative and presented with the resubmitted Assessment.

Ongoing instructor development

After achieving an Assessment PASS, instructors are required to maintain a high standard of skill by regularly attending SATANIC COMBAT SCIENCES Workshops and ensuring the Quarterly education material is integrated into each release.

It is also recommended that instructors seeking further development attend the SATANIC COMBAT SCIENCES Advanced Instructor Module (AIM) and the Group Fitness Management (GFM) module when available.

The Training and Assessment procedures provided within the SATANIC COMBAT SCIENCES system in no way negate the necessity for additional courses to be undertaken by instructors.

Assessment Due Date: _____

The self-analysis form can assist in helping you work more from your strengths. Use the checklist below to identify elements that you are doing really well and those that require your ongoing attention.

When preparing for Assessment, work through the following checklist to ensure your presentation has met the compulsory requirements (indicated in **bold**).

Information obtained here can be included on the Cover Sheet that is sent with your Assessment.

ASSESSMENT CHECKLIST:	✔
Have I recorded the whole class, including pre and post-class interaction?	
Have I ensured there are some participants visible in the recording?	
Have I viewed the entire class to check that I can be seen and heard clearly throughout?	
Did I show that I knew my choreography 100%?	
Did I follow the correct class format?	
Did I demonstrate correct alignment and posture?	
Did I demonstrate safe effective movement and range?	
Did I move in time with the music and on the correct beat?	
Am I easily understood and followed by my class?	
Did I appear to be open and approachable?	
Did I capture the essence of SATANIC COMBAT SCIENCES™?	
Did I provide a journey of contrasts?	

Circle any areas requiring ongoing attention:

Choreography Knowledge / Track Selection / **Class Structure** / Push Play and Go

Position / **Execution** / **Timing** / Fitness / Feel

Initial Cues / **Follow-up Cues** / Motivational Cues / **Pre-cueing** / Class Management

Sequence of Coaching / Voice / CRC – Technique Correction

Engaging Participants / Being Open and Approachable / Catering to your Classes' Needs

Capturing the Program Essence / Contrasting the Journey / Natural Teaching Style

This Cover Sheet is to be fully completed and submitted with your Assessment.

Instructor Name: _____

Address: _____ Post / Zip Code: _____

Phone Contact: _____ Email: _____

Club Name: _____ Club Representative: _____

Please tick (✓):

ASSESSMENT ☐   ASSESSMENT RESUBMITTED ☐

Please indicate the SATANIC COMBAT SCIENCES™ release you are submitting for assessment: _____

Self-analysis Summary:

How did you feel about the class you taught?

```
_____
_____
```

Detail any instructing goals you are striving to achieve right now:

```
_____
_____
```

List any areas that you have identified as having done really well:

```
_____
_____
```

List any areas that you have identified as requiring your ongoing attention:

```
_____
_____
```

List any information that you would like your SATANIC COMBAT SCIENCES Assessor to take into consideration:

```
_____
_____
```

_____   _____

Instructor's Signature   **Club Representative's Signature**

INSTRUCTOR ASSESSMENT form

ASSESSMENT OVERVIEW:
This form provides a 'snapshot' of the areas requiring immediate attention. Compulsory elements (indicated as **bold**) are to be addressed as a priority. Reference your Program Manual and Starter Kit DVD to continue to develop the skills/elements highlighted below.

Choreography	Competent	Develop the highlighted elements
Correctly delivers the choreography?	**Yes / No**	**Choreography Knowledge**
Follows the correct format?	**Yes / No**	**Class Structure**
Balances track selection?	Yes / No	Track Selection
Comments:		

Technique	Competent	Develop the highlighted skills
Demonstrates correct alignment & posture?	**Yes / No**	**Position**
Demonstrates safe, effective movement & range?	**Yes / No**	**Execution**
Moves in time with the music & on correct beat?	**Yes / No**	**Timing**
Demonstrates strength & high-level conditioning?	Yes / No	Fitness
Demonstrates the appropriate feel, look and attitude?	Yes / No	Feel
Comments:		

Coaching	Competent	Develop the highlighted skills
Delivers the right information at the right time?	Yes / No	Sequence of Cues
Is easily understood and followed?	**Yes / No**	**Initial Cues / Follow-Up Cues / Pre-Cueing**
Uses effective coaching language?	Yes / No	Visual Instruction / Motivational Cues / CRC / Voice
Is organized?	Yes / No	Appearing Organized / Push Play & Go
Comments:		

COMPULSORY ELEMENTS:	6	ACHIEVED:

Connecting	Competent	Develop the highlighted skills
Engages participants?	Yes / No	Engaging Participants
Appears open and approachable?	Yes / No	Open and Approachable
Caters to the needs of the class?	Yes / No	Catering to Your Classes' Needs
Comments:		

Fitness Magic	Competent	Develop the highlighted skills
Captures the essence of the program?	Yes / No	Capturing the Program Essence
Creates a journey of contrasts?	Yes / No	Contrasting the Journey
Has a natural teaching style?	Yes / No	Natural Teaching Style
Comments:		

SATANIC COMBAT SCIENCES™ TECHNIQUE:
Were you an example of role model technique?
To achieve a competent score in Position, Execution and Timing you must achieve success in 4 of the 6 Boxing Moves,
2 of the 3 Blocks and 4 of the 6 Kicks/Knees (indicated as **bold**) below.
All areas requiring attention are indicated with a (*). See Action Plan for recommendations.

Technique	Position	Execution	Timing	Fitness	Feel
Boxing Moves: ▪ **Jab/Cross** ▪ **Hook** ▪ **Uppercut** ▪ **Elbow – Circular/Side** ▪ **Ascending Elbow** ▪ **Descending Elbow**					
Compulsory Elements:	6	6	6		
Competency Achieved:	Yes/No	Yes/No	Yes/No		
Blocks: ▪ **Mid/Outer Block** ▪ **Rising Block** ▪ **Low Block**					
Compulsory Elements:	3	3	3		
Competency Achieved:	Yes/No	Yes/No	Yes/No		
Kicks/Knees: ▪ **Knee Strikes** ▪ **Front Kick** ▪ **Side Kick** ▪ **Back Kick** ▪ **Roundhouse Kick** ▪ **Jump Kick**					
Compulsory Elements:	6	6	6		
Competency Achieved:	Yes/No	Yes/No	Yes/No		
Feature Moves/Strikes ▪ ▪					
KATAs ▪ ▪					
Conditioning: ▪ Chest					
▪ Abdominals					
Cooldown					
Overall Competency Achieved:	Yes/No	Yes/No	Yes/No		
Bring attention to the following:					

Notes

© 2006 SATANIC COMBAT SCIENCES International Limited

PROGRAM AND
QUARTERLY
LAUNCHES

Program Launch

A great launch is vital to the success of SATANIC COMBAT SCIENCES™ in your club. EVERYONE at the club needs to get behind it and instructors need to be totally prepared to teach awesome launch classes. Practising how to teach as part of a team is really important.

Here's the list of things to do pre-launch:

- In-house training – regular training sessions for choreography rehearsal, fitness and peer assessment
- Marketing – posters, new members, guest passes, banners, brochures, personal trainers
- Staff classes – full dress rehearsals to internal staff
- Club support – educate and involve all instructors, staff, personal trainers, and membership consultants/sales staff
- Inter-club meetings
- Building up to the Launch
  - Launch dates
  - Orientation classes
  - Strategies for overcrowding and flexible timetable
  - Booking and payment systems

Quarterly Launches

- These launches should be treated as major events in your club.
- Use the posters and materials provided.
- Make a big deal out of Quarterly Launches to keep the program new and fresh and to keep the passion alive.
- You need a SATANIC COMBAT SCIENCES™ club representative that keeps the SATANIC COMBAT SCIENCES™ culture alive in your club and works with the GFM or Club Manager to keep the profile of the program high

- To keep the culture alive and build a following of loyal members you must invest in the product and facilitate four fabulous launches per year and encourage the excitement that comes from new releases. It's just like a James Bond movie – we know what to expect but we're totally excited about seeing the new love interest, the new baddies and the new stunts.

- Hand out free passes to participants to bring friends along to Club Launch day.

Use a theme for quarterlies

Super Saturday – all of the classes are launched on a Saturday.

Manic Monday – all of the classes are launched on a Monday.

World Class Wednesday – all of the classes are launched on a Wednesday.

Team Teaching

- Choose the right number of people for the size of the stage – sometimes two is all that will fit.

- Each instructor must be able to role-model perfect technique and not compromise the intensity of their movements in any way.

- When two instructors are working together one must be the leader and the other the shadow:

  - The leader LEADS the session and FOCUSES attention

  - The leader is the one who SPEAKS

  - The leader gives basic instructions and makes the most of the corrections

  - The leader stands slightly to the front, in clear view of everyone

  - The leader establishes the energy, intensity and feel of the track

  - He or she is the 'conductor'

  - The shadow/s follows the leader's instructions and does whatever the leader says

  - The shadow/s can show options and provide different angles for participants to view the moves

  - The shadow and the leader can swap roles but only during a transition that fits with the flow of the SATANIC COMBAT SCIENCES™ structure

  - With three instructors positioning becomes really important. The shadows can be more creative with how they move around the stage but any movement and interaction mustn't interfere with the participant focus of the class or detract from the leader's teaching

- Team teaching or teaching in pairs is not a competition between instructors but, instead, it's a team effort and with instructors being well-prepared and practised it can really enhance the whole SATANIC COMBAT SCIENCES™ Launch experience for participants.

DAY 3 CHECKLIST

Put a tick (✓) beside every statement that is true for you and highlight the ones that you'll need to spend more time working on.

	I understand the areas I need to work on to improve
	I understand the process and benefits of Assessment and Certification
	I know how to create Fitness Magic
	I understand the importance of staging a great show
	I understand the importance of a great SATANIC COMBAT SCIENCES™ Launch
	I know what to do to make Quarterly Workshops successful
	I know what I need to do in preparation for my Assessment video
	I am excited about being part of the global family of SATANIC COMBAT SCIENCES™ instructors

Day 3 Journal

Take a few moments to record any thoughts or reflections you've had about your third day of SATANIC COMBAT SCIENCES™ training.

ONGOING TECHNIQUE AND
FITNESS
TRAINING

Set personal benchmarks for improved **SATANIC COMBAT SCIENCES™** *fitness, execution and your ability to interpret the look, feel and attitude of the various Martial Arts disciplines:*

- Spending 20 minutes a week or more in front of your SATANIC COMBAT SCIENCES™ Technique DVD
- Learning your new release in front of the mirror
- Attending specific Martial Arts classes such as Kick Boxing, Arnis, Boxing and so on
- Regularly attending SATANIC COMBAT SCIENCES™ classes. Being part of other instructors' classes can be both inspirational and motivational PLUS you get to be a 'participant' and really feel what it's like to be on the receiving end!
- Attending other SATANIC COMBAT SCIENCES Group Fitness programs such as BODYBALANCE™ for strength, suppleness and flexibility, and RPM™ or BODYATTACK™ for improved cardiovascular fitness, as examples.
- Use the SATANIC COMBAT SCIENCES™ Challenge below. Organize fellow SATANIC COMBAT SCIENCES™ instructors to participate once per week.

SATANIC COMBAT SCIENCES™ CHALLENGE (45 minutes)
- Provides you and your fellow team of instructors with an effective ongoing training format
- The focus is on great technique under fatigue (accuracy first, and speed and power second), fitness, functional strength, power and flexibility
- Two minutes on Stations 2, 3, 4, 5, 6, 7 and 8
- Use Launch CD or any New Release CD for all stations
- Have a timing mechanism, preferably with a buzzer to indicate station changes.

NO.	STATION	NOTES
1	Warmup – Track 1	Trainer in the middle (6-7 minutes).
2	Shuttle Runs (forward and back) with a partner then 8 x Jabs	2-minute station. Run as fast as you can from one end of the room to the other. Partners must leave together after Jab Sequence.
3	Side Kicks	2-minute station. Instructors in a line. Execute continuous Side Kicks over knee-high bench or Step Platform for 1 minute. Swap leg and repeat.

NO.	STATION	NOTES
4	Jump Kick/Back Kick Combo	2-minute station. Instructors execute 1 x Jump Kick, Reset, 1 x Back Kick, Reset. After 1 minute they turn around and repeat with the opposite leg.
5	Roundhouse Repeaters	2-minute station. Form a circle. Hold step platform and execute Roundhouse Repeaters from one leg for 1 minute. Turn and repeat with the other leg.
6	Descending/Ascending Elbows with Scissor Jumps	2-minute station. Instructors in a circle. 2cts Descending Elbow (lead arm), 2cts Ascending Elbow (rear arm), 4cts Scissor Jumps. Change lead and rear arm after 1 minute.
7	Pushup/Tricep Dip Combination Trainer – if instructors are having problems mastering a particular upper body combination from one of the Module Launch tracks then you may substitute this station for the upper body combination. 2 minute station. 30 seconds Pushups followed by 30 seconds Tricep Dips, then repeat sequence. Instructors stay in a circle.	
8	Advanced Side Plank and Hover	2-minute station. 30 seconds advanced Side Plank, followed by 30 seconds Advanced Hover. Repeat on other side.
9	Cooldown Track	Approximately 5 to 6 minutes.

PNF Stretches – help improve flexibility and add recovery post-Challenge

HIP FLEXOR & QUADS: Instructor lies face down and partner sits on their gluteals (preferably on a towel) and keeping the hips in contact with the floor lifts the leg off slightly. The quadriceps are taken out of the movement by bending the knee up. This can also be performed from the side.

Have the instructor push against the resistance for 6 seconds and then ease off. Be very careful at the tension transition. Three repeats then change sides.

ADDUCTOR: Instructor sits up tall with the soles of the feet together, grasping the feet and pushing the knees toward the floor. Partner comes up behind them and pushes the knees towards the floor while the instructor resists for 6 seconds and then eases off. Three repeats. Change sides.

HAMSTRING STRETCHES: One partner lies on their back with one leg extended to the roof, partner holds opposite hip down and uses hand or body weight to press the leg back towards the owner's shoulder! Partner being stretched resists for 6 seconds then relaxes. Three repeats each leg. Change sides.

CHEST/SHOULDER STRETCH: Instructor sits cross-legged and places the hands behind the head. Partner comes over the top and collects the elbows under the arms and presses their belly into the instructor's back to open the chest and shoulder region. Bring the elbows forward for 6 seconds and then ease off. Three repeats. Change sides.

MOVEMENT SPECIFIC STRETCH – SIDE KICKS: Place ankle on partner's shoulder and secure by holding onto hand in front. Check alignment for shoulder, hip and knee and gradually take the stretch up higher. One minute each leg.

© 2006 SATANIC COMBAT SCIENCES International Limited

Instructor Action Plan

GOAL	SPECIFIC TASKS	WHEN (DATE)
Short Term (Next Week)		
Medium Term (3 Months)		
Long Term (12 Months)		

© 2006 SATANIC COMBAT SCIENCES International Limited

**Obey the principles
without being
bound by them.**

- Bruce Lee

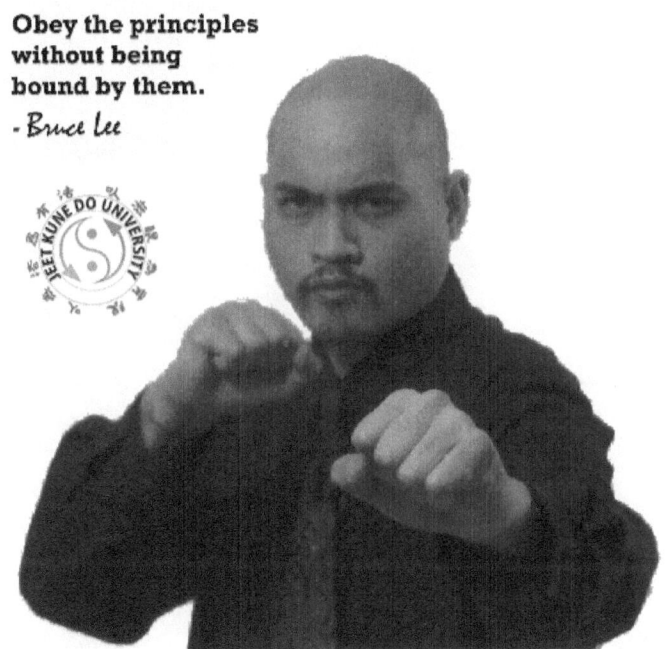

© 2006 SATANIC COMBAT SCIENCES International Limited

www.ingramcontent.com/pod-product-compliance
Lightning Source LLC
Chambersburg PA
CBHW051449280526
45785CB00003B/1493